A Playbook Between

The Memory Challenged Client & The Caregiver

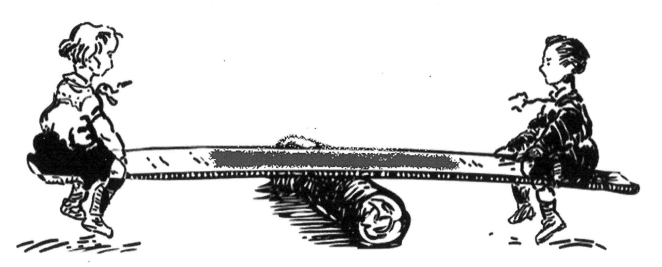

By

Beth Lord, OTR/L, GCFP, SFP

ISBN: 10:1-62269-010-9

ISBN-13: 978-1-62269-010-7

Other Books by Beth Lord

Points of Consciousness from The Camino

Finding Otis

The House On 16th Ave. N.E.

La Dolce Vita a Villa Picalò/Living The Sweet Life At Villa Picalò

ASMR:Autonomous Sensory Meridian Response

Five Easy Steps For Turning Your Stories Into Books

DEDICATION

To Mary, Peter, Bob & Linda, and the team of caregivers who have given their all for Peter to have a vibrant daily life worth living.

To Lou & Jackie who are an extraordinary dynamic duo who have seen each other through thick and thin.

To caregiving and caregivers in general. It's not about control but a balancing of giving and receiving in our minds, hearts and movement.

CONTENTS

Acknowledgements   vii

Caregiving   1

In Doing These Lessons   3

Introduction by Beth Lord, OTR/L, GCFP, SFP   5

The Playbook

Affirmations   11

Balls   15

Be The Amazing You That You Are   19

Be Present   23

Body Talk and Tapping Out The Cortices   27

Brain Exercises   29

Breath   47

Bubbles   49

Calendars & Cues   51

Celebration   53

Certificate of Amazingness and Approval   55

Comfort Zone   57

Checklists For Daily Activities   65

Color   69

Communication   75

Compassion   79

Feelings   81

The "Fight or Flight" Response   85

Focus   89

Forgiveness   91

Going Fishing   93

Going Out In The Community   96

Healing   99

Inspiration   103

Laughter   105

Living With A Head Injury   109

The Playbook

Lumosity	113
Make Yourself Comfortable	115
Meditation	121
Memory - Brain, Gut, Muscle and Heart	125
Memory Boards	127
Movement	129
Music, Songs, Sing, Sounds, Hum & Chant	131
Nourish	133
Novelty	135
Organizing and Simplifying	137
Our Bios	139
Pain	141
Play	143
Read To Each Other	145
Routines	147
Smell	149
Start Your Story	151
Walk	153
What Motivates You? *Maslow's Hierarchy of Needs*	157
What Is Your Story For The Day?	159
Whole Brain Involvement	161
When I Get Mad I Talk To My Hand	163
Writing Poems	165
You Matter	171

vi

ACKNOWLEDGEMENTS

To the people who have been a part of my life who have blessed me with their love of care, healing and wholeness. Their determination to have a great life has inspired this playbook.

What Do You Want To Learn From This Playbook?

Client:

_____

_____

_____

_____

_____

_____

_____

Caregiver:

_____

_____

_____

_____

_____

_____

_____

What is the word you are breathing into who you are?

Client's Word: _____

Caregiver's Word: _____

CAREGIVING

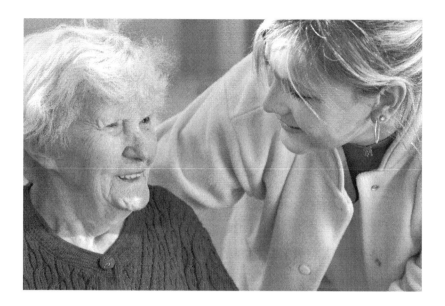

…..There are basically two problems caregivers have. First, they treat the person like an inanimate object, instead of engaging their nervous system to cooperate with them. Second, they really don't know how the body works, how it's connected, and what's the easiest way to move oneself or another person ……

…improving the quality of the contact and the relationship is desperately needed because people get so frazzled… You know, caregivers get sick and die sometimes before their charge does because they are so run ragged….

….There is some staggering number of people in the United States who are caring for family members, and that will only increase as the Baby Boom generation ages. Most of us are likely to pass through this role sometime in our lives, plus many more people will be needed to do caregiving work in a professional capacity, so it is an enormous need, a huge population and very stressed, very much in need of support….

Excepts from

Bringing Feldenkrais Care to Caregivers

3/31/2015

In Touch interviews Nancy Gayle Judson, GCFP and Annie Gottlieb, Member Trainee

In Touch Spring 2015

How Do You Feel?

Caregiver: _____

Client: _____

In Doing These Lessons

If writing is difficult for you, record your thoughts and information on a recorder, iPhone, iPad or smart phone, so you play your thoughts back to yourself. These expressed thoughts and conversations are the bridge builders between you and The Caregiver or you and The Memory Challenged Client (called "client" from now on). Using this playbook creates a positive impact on both parties because these lessons rejuvenate you and supports a dynamic balance between The Caregiver and The Client. Enjoy these adventures into yourself. - Beth

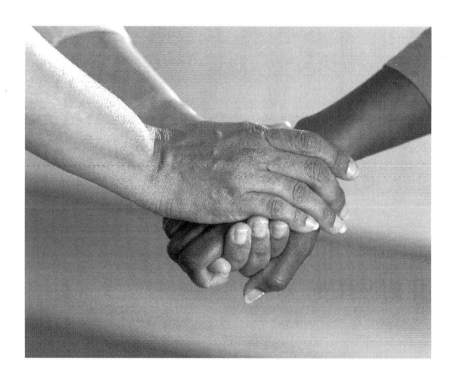

Are We Ready To Begin?

Introduction by Beth Lord, OTR/L, GCFP, SFP

I have been an Occupational Therapist for over 30 years. Occupational Therapy is defined by the World Federation of Occupational Therapists as the following:

> Occupational therapy is a client-centered health profession concerned with promoting health and well-being through occupation. The primary goal of occupational therapy is to enable people to participate in the activities of everyday life. (WFOT 2012)

I began my career working two jobs. One was in the school systems in a county nearby Chicago, and the other one was for a home health agency. It was a perfect balance for me because I worked with children in the schools and saw adults and older adults in their homes. There were many different clients, conditions, and needs that had to be evaluated to see what was the biggest problem area I could provide achievable goals with my services. I realized this was easy to do when I listened to what my clients and their families needed. My listening to clients and caregivers helped them build a healthy foundation for creating their support system for health, wholeness and happiness.

Margot Heiniger and Shirley Randolph spoke in my last year studying to be an OT at the U. of Kansas, and I bought their book: "*Neurophysiological Concepts In Human Behavior - The Tree of Learning*." I took extra classes to learn how to test for *Sensory-Integration Dysfunction*. This dysfunction had been researched and developed by *A Jean Ayres Ph.D.*, who was an Occupational Therapist and a developmental psychologist. I went to San Diego every summer for ten years and listened to *Dr. Josephine C Moore, Ph.D.* talk about the application of neurophysiological concepts in everyday life. **Neurophysiology was my gateway into a possibility of gaining more health and wholeness for someone**. If I could explain a technique or a tool that could benefit the nervous system, it became part of my toolkit.

I easily moved into a private practice because people saw that I was different, and they wanted to work with me or have their kids work with me. Their faith in me did not get wasted as I constantly researched possibilities and listened to their needs. This passion within me has never stopped. I DO believe that it is sacred to work with people and their families who are vulnerable, going through trauma, tragedy, and transition. Respecting these folks by listening to them is a great start for them believing in themselves and moving forward.

I trained with **Dr. John Upledger**, who was the founder of **Cranial-Sacral Therapy**. I trained with **John Barnes**, who is a physical therapist and one of the leading founders of **Myofascial Release**. I worked 1:1 with clients in their homes, my office or with institutions in a contract situation when they wanted my expertise. One of the contracts I worked with was a "test pilot" Holistic Mental Health Program in Chicago for people who had a manic-depressive disorder. I was excited to be on this team because there were many innovators and visionaries on it. One of the practitioners was **James Kavanaugh**, a former Catholic Priest who came to fame in 1067 with his controversial bestseller "**A Modern Priest Looks At His Outdated Church**." He was also a psychologist and a poet. I learned, from him, the therapeutic importance of writing poetry and your stories for self-expression and healing.

I treated a young girl who had Cerebral Palsy. This young girl also worked with **Anat Baniel**. Anat is one of the original Feldenkrais Practitioners who went on to develop **The Anat Baniel Method** and wrote about it in her book, "**The Nine Essentials For Lifelong Vitality - Move Into Life With The Anat Baniel Method**." Anat and I would work together with this young girl. We were both doing great things, but I wanted what Anat was doing. Anat is a gifted mentor, healer, teacher, practitioner and clear about how wonderful this method is and told me, flat out, I should become a **Feldenkrais Practitioner**. The year was 1988 and we were planning a move from Chicago to Seattle. It just so happened that **Jeff Haller** was offering his first training to become a Feldenkrais Practitioner in Seattle the month after we moved there. I took the training.

The training was for two months every year for four years. We were on our backs exploring movement the entire training time to become more aware of how our mind created our movement possibilities. We had amazing Feldenkrais Trainers besides Jeff, including **Jerry Karzen** and **Ruthy Alon** helping us feel the connection between movement and our minds. They taught us that our movement could be slow and gentle - filled with the possibilities of making ourselves more comfortable. One of the women who was in my training had a brain aneurysm years later and wrote about her experience. Her name is **Judith Marcus,** and her book is: "**Uncoiling - A Memoir Of Anxiety, Aneurysm, and Renewal**."

I started my Therapeutic Toy Catalog business, **Play With Success,** saw clients of all sorts, wrote the book, "**Play With Success,**" and raised three girls. I played with success with my growing girls and took to heart **The Feldenkrais Method**®. I practiced these methods and continued to gather tools and techniques to strengthen brain development, rehabilitation and wholeness within one's self. I exhibited my therapeutic toys at **The American Holistic Medical Association Conference** for three years. I was able to listen to talks from people like **Dr. Deepak Chopra, Dr. Christine Northrup, Carolyn Myss and Patch Adams.** It was a fantastic learning opportunity for me and my **"Play With Success"** ideas. At first, Doctors would look at my table and would want to know why I was there. Why were toys at a Holistic Medical Conference? I'd talk about the power of touch and play as therapeutic and healing - an inroad, to our child-like wonder, laughter and fun. When we play, we have an opportunity to be in the present moment. I was there, playing with toys and encouraging doctors, to touch the toys and explore. Even the holistic doctors were hesitant to play. But little by little, someone, would touch a toy and then, that would lead another one to touch a toy and soon, there were many people playing, laughing and being in the present moment.

I have been a Feldenkrais Practitioner for over 25 years now. I had my toy catalog company for over eight years. I worked at a Traumatic Head Injury Rehab Center as The OT Director. While I was there, I met Lou, who suffered a stroke. He never went back to work, but he did form a head injury support group that is still going strong twenty years later. Caregiver support was another group formed because the need for caregivers to have support is critical. The relationship between The Caregiver and The Client is a balancing act that is always in motion.

I met Peter over 14 years ago and started working with him as his Occupational Therapist and his Feldenkrais Practitioner. But first, I balanced his stress reactions and his **"fight or flight" responses.** These responses made him angry and aggressive with the caregiver or fleeing into the bathroom for long periods of time because he was confused in his memory. We set up memory cues to decrease these responses, schedules so he had consistency and checklists so he could see what he had done during the day. We made sure we were having fun while teaching him step by step behavior that balances the "fight or flight responses" and builds success and happiness in daily life.

Motivation is different for everyone but we made sure we reinforced what Peter wanted to do if it was reasonable. His Dad and Linda (his step-mom) are his biggest advocates, then and now, as they help Peter live a full life. His team from U. of Washington Medical Center helps him get his medication under control while his home team works on his motivation. Peter has positive support and we communicate with each other for further support. Peter exercises, eats healthy, is out and about in community, does fabulous pottery and has balanced his **"Fight or Flight" reactions. He has a great life.**

"The fight or flight" response is explained later in this book, but this is important for both the caregiver and the client to know about for daily life. It's about minimizing stress reactions to change in daily life. If someone is feeling safe, secure and comfortable, then this reaction is minimized. The focus of the day can embrace partnering with each other and share healthy attitudes, behaviors and feelings for both the client and the caregiver.

I listened to the caregivers and spent a great deal of time with them because they WERE influencing Peter. Every moment of possibility is every moment of possibility, and *I wanted the caregivers to know that THEY ARE THE POWER of impact*. This playbook has many lessons in it that Peter's team of caregivers and me have worked on with Peter. The learning exercises have been created for both the caregiver and client so they can work together in a positive, balanced way.

Neuroplasticity is a happening word. It means our brains can form new connections and learn new information. Even as we get older and have trauma, brain, and memory loss. I would encourage you to look up *Norman Doidge, M.D.* because he has written two books on the subject *"The Brain That Changes Itself "*and *"The Brain's Way of Healing."*

 It's vital that the client's environment is set up for success. Pictures of the client involved in his life around the home. Pictures involving her and her family. A calendar of what's going on in his/her life (in an easy place to reference like on the refrigerator), daily checklists, pictures and simple bios of the caregivers. Even if the caregiver is a husband, wife or other family member, that bio and picture need to be up there for an appropriate boundary marker between their personal and professional lives. If a family member is volunteering to be a caregiver, it is still a profession that the client has to respect. The boundaries between personal and professional caregiving is a slippery slope. Clear boundaries help everyone involved.

A clean, simple and organized home makes a big difference as a healthy, therapeutic milieu. Set up work stations that the client can go to for memory work, creative work, cooking and other activities that are interesting to the client. As much as possible, the client needs to participate in activities that make his house a home because she is part of that home. He is part of the home.

Caregivers face "burn out" and we'd like to head them off at the pass so they keep their motivation for this kind of work. This playbook is designed to be an easy tool to support caregivers and clients.

The client needs to know his story. If he has trouble knowing his story, then it is important to nourish him with his story on a daily (as you can) basis. Knowing how the caregiver feels and how the memory challenged client feels helps the day be supportive. Because once you know the feelings and can express those feelings (in a helpful, not a hurtful way), the feelings can move along and become another feeling. So here then, is a playbook of possibilities for rejuvenation, health and wholeness for the caregiver and client. These lessons are meant to be copied and used to be of help to all concerned so no worries about ©. Use this playbook in this way to support you. Write back to me with suggestions and how you're using this playbook. And let me know your stories!

When you buy five or more printed books, the purchase price goes down to $ 9.99 so you can spread the word and keep the extra money for yourself or give it away. It's my way of appreciating what you're doing for me.

Thank-You!

Most Warmly,

Beth

Beth Lord, OTR/L, GCFP, SFP

www.bethlord.com

beth@bethlord.com

Seattle, WA. June 22, 2015

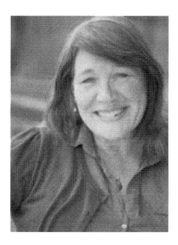

What Tingles Your Fancy & Makes You Feel Like You're Having Fun.

Life is Good Because You're Alive!

Caregiver:

_____

_____

_____

_____

_____

Client:

_____

_____

_____

_____

_____

Affirmations

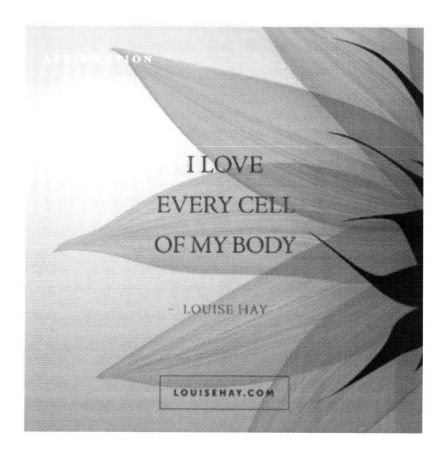

You ARE what you say.

Thoughts are affirming in both a positive and negative way.

STOP and pay attention to the words that are coming out of your mouth.

If you begin to notice your words, you begin to have choice in what you are choosing to say.

• The goal is to accept yourself.

• Bring in the positive thoughts and your words will be positive too.

• Affirmations create the environment you are working or living in.
   Positive thoughts + Positive Words = A Healthy Environment.

Both caregiver and client can compile their favorite affirmations to say to each other as they begin their day or during the day or upon retiring. Both caregiver and the client are more unified as a positive team when they say their affirmations to each other.

You can make up your own affirmations or find examples on these websites that say what you want to say.

Lesson One
Check out these affirmation web-sites and bookmark your favorite ones.
These bookmarks can be positive support for both the caregiver and the client.

1.   http://www.louisehay.com/affirmations/

2.   http://www.prolificliving.com/100-positive-affirmations/

3.   http://www.self-help-and-self-development.com/affirmations.html

4.   http://www.creativeaffirmations.com/list-of-affirmations.html

5.   http://tinybuddha.com/blog/how-to-change-your-mind-and-your-life-by-using-affirmations/

6.   http://www.vitalaffirmations.com/affirmations.htm#.Vty43ZMrKi5

7.   https://www.pinterest.com/superkp/positive-affirmations/

8.   http://www.chopra.com/ccl/7-affirmations-for-self-healing

9.   http://www.yogananda-srf.org/Affirmations.aspx#.Vty5b5MrKi5

10.   https://www.powerofpositivity.com/

Lesson One (con't)

Caregiver - Which sites are your favorite?

_____

_____

_____

Client - Which sites are your favorite?

_____

_____

_____

Lesson Two

Top 5 Affirmations you are going to say on a daily basis.

Caregiver

1._____

2._____

3._____

4._____

5._____

Top 5 Affirmations you are going to say on a daily basis.

Client

1._____

2._____

3._____

4._____

5._____

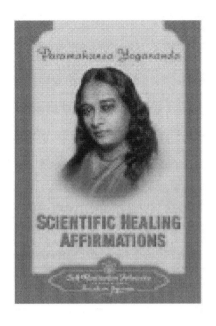

"As one uses different affirmations, his attitude of mind should change; for example, **WILL** affirmations should be accompanied by strong determination; **FEELING** affirmations by devotion, REASON affirmation by clear understanding. When healing others, select an affirmation that is suitable to the cognitive, imaginative, emotional, or thoughtful temperament of your patient. In all affirmations intensity of attention comes first, but continuity and repetition mean a great deal, too. Impregnate your affirmations with devotion, will, and faith, intensely and repeatedly, unmindful of the results, which will come naturally as the fruit of your labors."

- Paramahansa Yogananda
Scientific Healing Affirmations

It is most effective to practice affirmations immediately after awakening in the morning or just before going to sleep at night. Before beginning an affirmation, it is important to sit in the correct meditation posture, on a chair or firm surface. The spine should be held erect, and the eyes closed, concentrating on the medulla oblongata at the back of the neck.

Free the mind from restless thoughts and worries.

- *http://www.yogananda-srf.org/Affirmations.aspx#.VVMMD6b8QoV*

Balls

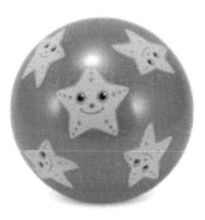

Balls are such an easy way to have fun. Get a simple, soft ball which can be found in any toy or drug store or ordered. You can choose the size that best.
meets your needs. It is a lovely activity getting you connected to each other.

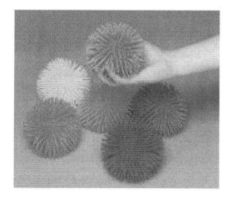

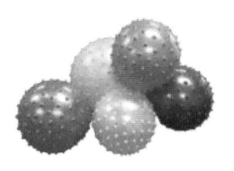

Smart Sheep Wool Dryer Balls Can Be Used For The Softness Factor.

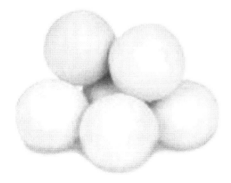

Lesson One

Sit down at a comfortable distance from one another so that both of you can catch the ball with two hands. Decide on the times you are going to catch it.

5x's. 10x's. 25x's.

Work to increase how many times you catch it.

- Further the distance between you.

- **Do the same activity but clap before you catch the ball. This is a great way to practice attention. It's also a memory enhancer as you need to remember clapping before catching the ball. Laughing, forgiving dropped balls and having fun.**

Lesson Two

Do the same thing but catch the ball with only your right hand. Decide on the times you both are going to catch it. 5x's. 10x's. 25x's.

Work to increase how many times you both catch it.

Lesson Three

Do the same thing but catch the ball with only your left hand. Decide on the times you are going to catch it.

5x's. 10x's. 25x's.

Work to increase how many times you both catch it.

Lesson Four

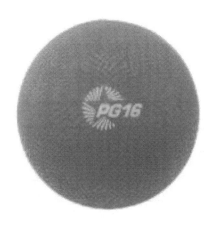

Stand up at a comfortable distance from one another so that you catch the ball with two hands. Decide on the times you are catching it.

5x's. 10x's. 25x's.

Work to increase how many times you catch it.

Further the distance between you.

- **Do the same activity but clap before you catch the ball. This is a great way to practice attention. It's also a memory enhancer as you need to remember clapping before catching the ball. Laughing, forgiving dropped balls and having fun.**

Balls

Lesson Five

Go outside and throw the ball against the garage or brick wall or some strong exterior that isn't near windows or doors to be broken and throw the ball against it and catch it. See how many times you can do this without dropping the ball.

Lesson Six

Go outside and throw the ball up in the air and catch it. See how many times you can do this without dropping the ball.

Lesson Seven

Go outside and throw the ball down to the ground and catch it when it pops up. See how many times you can do this without dropping the ball.

Lesson Eight

For this you'll need a smaller tennis-sized ball if you've been using a larger ball. Sit close enough to pass the ball to one another. The first person starts with the ball in his left hand and passes it to his right hand. With his right hand, he passes it to the other person's left hand. That person passes the ball from his left hand to his right hand. From his right hand, he passes it to the other person's left hand and so on and so on until you don't want to do it anymore.

Name some of your Ball Activities

Client:

1._____

2._____

3._____

4._____

5._____

6._____

7._____

8._____

Caregiver:

1._____

2._____

3._____

4._____

5._____

6._____

7._____

8._____

Be The Amazing You That You Are

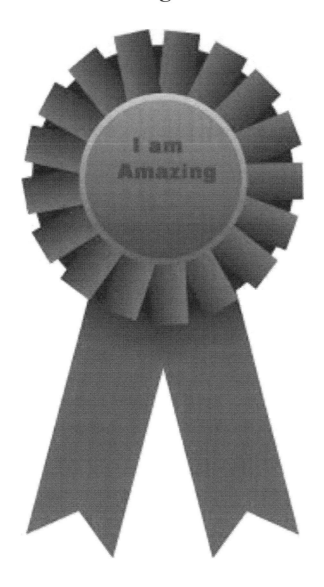

You don't have to do anything but be who you are.
You are amazing because you are.

Be The Amazing You That You Are

Lesson One.

Pay attention to you.
There is no one else like you.

Client: Tell your caregiver 3 things you find extraordinary about him/her.

1._____

2._____

3._____

Caregiver: Tell your cared for client 3 things you find extraordinary about him/her.

1._____

2._____

3._____

A). Say them aloud to each other.

B). Discuss how you observe these things in each other.

This relationship is mutually reinforcing with one another. The caregiver can cue the client, and the client can cue the caregiver. The teeter totter in the relationship can be balancing for both people involved.

Be The Amazing You That You Are

Lesson Two.

Pay attention to you and feel that you are amazing because you are unique in who you are. There is no one else like you.

Client: Write down 3 things you find extraordinary about yourself.

1._____

2._____

3._____

Caregiver: Write down 3 things you find extraordinary about yourself.

1._____

2._____

3._____

A). Say them aloud to each other.

B). Discuss how you came to these observations within yourself.

Be The Amazing You That You Are

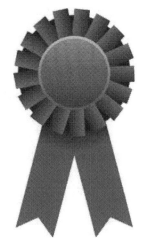

Lesson Three

Keep Track of All The Amazing Things You Do

Client

_____

_____

_____

_____

_____

_____

Caregiver

_____

_____

_____

_____

_____

_____

Be Present

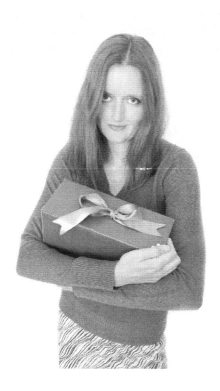

Being in the present moment requires focus in our mind, heart, stomach and body for that's where our energy is. We have to talk to these centers and connect them to us. It is helpful if we stop what we are doing so we can pay attention to this new skill we are learning.

We start in a quiet place to feel the chatter going on in our brain so we can stop it.

Yes, we stop the mind chatter so we have a sense of who we are and where we are.

If I have chatter going on in my brain then I am not paying attention to the present.

I am not with you and I am not with myself. If I stop the chatter in my mind

then I have a greater chance to know me. I have a greater chance to know you.

Lesson One

Spend 1 minute paying attention to what's going on now.
Then write about it and discuss what went on for both of you.

Caregiver:

_____

_____

_____

Client:

_____

_____

_____

Lesson Two

Spend 5 minutes paying attention to what's going on now.
Then write about it and discuss what went on for both of you.

Caregiver:

_____

_____

_____

Client:

_____

_____

_____

Be Present

Lesson Three

Spend 15 minutes paying attention to what's going on now.
Then write about it and discuss what went on for both of you.

Caregiver:

_____

_____

_____

Client:

_____

_____

_____

Lesson Four

Spend 30 minutes paying attention to what's going on now.
Then write about it and discuss what went on for both of you.

Caregiver:

_____

_____

_____

Client:

_____

_____

_____

Be Present

Further Resources.

https://www.psychologytoday.com/blog/enlightened-living/201106/5-steps-being-present

http://www.spiritualityandpractice.com/practices/practices.php?id=3

http://tinybuddha.com/blog/5-lessons-about-being-present-freedom-is-where-my-feet-are/

http://presentliving.com/whatisbeingpresent/

http://zenhabits.net/mindful/

http://www.peterrussell.com/SpiritAwake/now.php

Body Talk and Tapping Out The Cortices

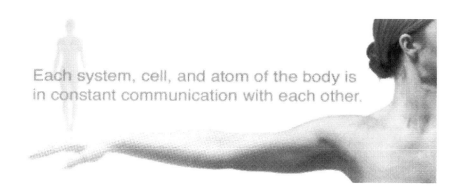

Each system, cell, and atom of the body is in constant communication with each other.

BodyTalk was developed by John Veltheim, D.C., B.Ac., CBI, SrCBI, CBI, ATI, BAT, when he had some compromising health issues and nothing was helping him. You can read his story here.

https://www.bodytalksystem.com/practitioners/details.cfm?id=381

I took the certification process of Body Talk and I like the techniques it offers in helping a person understand their body better. The following information was taken off their website. If you are interested in learning more there is a lot of information to be found on their website as well as on youtube videos. You can also find a certified practitioner through this organization's website as well. https://www.bodytalksystem.com

"BodyTalk: Healthcare designed by your body. BodyTalk is WholeHealthcare ™

The Body/Talk System seeks to address the "whole person". This means that no aspect of the human psyche can be overlooked, be it emotional, physical or environmental. In BodyTalk, we have developed a whole-healthcare system that supports and promotes the well being of any person, animal, or plant.

As Whole-Healthcare ™, BodyTalk understands the profound influence the psychology of the body has on our health. Instead of focusing on the symptom, BodyTalk finds the underlying causes of illness by addressing the whole-person and their whole-story.

Body Talk and Tapping Out The Cortices

The BodyTalk techniques provide insights to the areas of your body that need attention. What might seem like an obvious problem to you is not necessary the one your body wants to address first.

This is the beauty of BodyTalk. It respects the body's own needs and determines your body's priorities for healing. Then with the use of a variety of non-invasive techniques. BodyTalkers refocus your body's natural healing response to establish better communication within the body.

Tapping Out The Cortices

This technique is very simple for you to learn, and it helps to revitalize the brain. The BodyTalk Association feels so strongly about it that they show you how to do this in a video. All you need to do is go here and watch the video.

https://www.bodytalksystem.com/learn/access/cortices.cfm

Brain Exercises

Lesson One:

How many words can you make out of Mississippi

Client   **Caregiver**

_____   _____

_____   _____

_____   _____

_____   _____

_____   _____

_____   _____

_____   _____

Brain Exercises

Lesson Two:

Upside-Down Reading.

Choose an article from a newspaper or magazine. Hold it upside down and read it until your brain gets tired. Increase the length you do this until you get to 5 minutes.

	Client	Caregiver
One Minute	_____	_____
Two Minutes	_____	_____
Three Minutes	_____	_____
Four Minutes	_____	_____
Five Minutes	_____	_____

Brain Exercises

Lesson Three:

Scan an article and cross out:

	Client	**Caregiver**
All the s's.	_____	_____
All the b's.	_____	_____
All the t's.	_____	_____
All the a's.	_____	_____
All the m's.	_____	_____

Brain Exercises

Lesson Four:

Write a short paragraph on the most important event that happened in your life and then read your paragraphs to each other.

Client

_____

_____

_____

_____ .

Caregiver

_____

_____

_____

_____ .

Brain Exercises

Lesson Five:

Say the months in chronological order. Then work together to get the months in alphabetical order. Take turns reading the months in alphabetical order.

Months	**Alphabetical Order**
January	_____
February	_____
March	_____
April	_____
May	_____
June	_____
July	_____
August	_____
September	_____
October	_____
November	_____
December	_____

What is your favorite month and why?

What is your favorite season and why?

Brain Exercises

Lesson Six:

Client   **Caregiver**

_____ _____   Count out loud by tens up to 100 as fast as you can.

_____ _____   Count backward by tens up to 100 as fast as you can.

_____ _____   Count out loud by twos up to 100 as fast as you can.

_____ _____   Count backward by twos from 100 to zero.

_____ _____   Count out loud by fives up to 100 as fast as you can.

_____ _____   Count backward by fives up to 100 as fast as you can.

Lesson Seven:

Drawing circles at the same time with both your right hand and left hand.
Color the circles in.

Client

Caregiver

Brain Exercises

Lesson Eight:

Beside each letter, write a word that begins with that letter that is related to you. Say each word out loud.

	Client	Caregiver
A	_____	_____
B	_____	_____
C	_____	_____
D	_____	_____
E	_____	_____
F	_____	_____
G	_____	_____
H	_____	_____
I	_____	_____
J	_____	_____
K	_____	_____
L	_____	_____

Brain Exercises

M   _____   _____

N   _____   _____

O   _____   _____

P   _____   _____

Q   _____   _____

R   _____   _____

S   _____   _____

T   _____   _____

U   _____   _____

V   _____   _____

W   _____   _____

X   _____   _____

Y   _____   _____

Z   _____   _____

Brain Exercises

Lesson Nine:

Write a paragraph or two about you that uses these words.

Client

_____

_____

_____

_____

_____

_____

_____

_____

Caregiver

_____

_____

_____

_____

_____

_____

_____

_____

_____

Brain Exercises

Lesson Ten:

Timelines.

Write down the events you remember up to that year and continue until you finish to the age you are at now.

---

5   10   15   20   25   30   35   40   45   50   55   60   65   70   75   80   90   95   100

Client:

Up to 5 years: _____, _____, _____, _____,

Caregiver: _____, _____, _____, _____,

Client:

Up to 10 years: _____, _____, _____, _____,

Caregiver: _____, _____, _____, _____,

Client:

Up to 15 years: _____, _____, _____, _____,

Caregiver: _____, _____, _____, _____,

Client:

Up to 20 years: _____, _____, _____, _____,

Caregiver: _____, _____, _____, _____,

Client:

Up to 25 years: _____, _____, _____, _____,

Caregiver: _____, _____, _____, _____,

Brain Exercises

Client:

Up to 30 years: _____, _____, _____, _____,

Caregiver: _____, _____, _____, _____,

Up to 30 years: _____, _____, _____, _____,

Client:

Up to 40 years: _____, _____, _____, _____,

Caregiver: _____, _____, _____, _____,

Client:

Up to 50 years: _____, _____, _____, _____,

Caregiver: _____, _____, _____, _____,

Client:

Up to 60 years: _____, _____, _____, _____,

Caregiver: _____, _____, _____, _____,

Client:

Up to 70 years: _____, _____, _____, _____,

Caregiver: _____, _____, _____, _____,

Client:

Up to 80 years: _____, _____, _____, _____,

Caregiver: _____, _____, _____, _____,

Brain Exercises

Client:

Up to 90 years: _____, _____,_____,_____,

Caregiver: _____, _____,_____,_____,

Client:

Up to 1000 years: _____, _____,_____,_____,

Caregiver: _____, _____,_____,_____,

Caregiver: Please feel free to put any extra events down here.

_____

_____

_____

_____

_____

Client: Please feel free to put any extra events down here.

_____

_____

_____

_____

_____

Brain Exercises

Lesson Eleven:

Brainstorming - solving real life problems.

1. How do we listen to each other?

Client and Caregiver:
Pick a project or a task that needs to get done and see what you can come up with as a team.

_____

_____

_____

_____

_____

_____

2. What do we do to support each other when one or both of us are having a bad day?

_____

_____

_____

_____

_____

_____

Brain Exercises

3. How do we recognize when each other is "tired" so we can "let go" and let relaxation happen instead of negative behavior escalating?

_____

_____

_____

_____

_____

_____

4. Other real life problems we need to work on.

_____

_____

_____

_____

_____

_____

Brain Exercises

Lesson Twelve:

Work together and finish these proverbs and put the meaning of it underneath the phrase. If you get stuck, all the information can be found on this website:

http://www.phrasemix.com/collections/the-50-most-important-english-proverbs

1. "The squeaky wheel _____."

    Meaning: _____

2. "Better late _____."

    Meaning: _____

3. "A picture is worth _____."

    Meaning: _____

4. "A watched pot _____."

    Meaning: _____

5. "Actions speak _____."

    Meaning: _____

Brain Exercises

6. "Don't bite the _____."

   Meaning: _____

7. "There's no time _____."

   Meaning: _____

8. "Two heads are _____."

   Meaning: _____

9. "You can lead a horse to water, _____."

   Meaning: _____

10. "Two wrongs _____."

   Meaning: _____

11. "When the going gets tough, _____."

   Meaning: _____

Brain Exercises

12. "People who live in glass houses _____."

Meaning: _____

13. "No man is _____."

Meaning: _____

14. "Birds of a feather _____."

Meaning: _____

15. "There's no place _____."

Meaning: _____

16. "Practice makes _____."

Meaning: _____

17. "Too many cooks _____."

Meaning: _____

Brain Exercises

18. "If you can't beat 'em, _____."

Meaning: _____

19. "One man's trash is _____."

Meaning: _____

Your Own:

Caregiver:

" _____."

Meaning: _____

" _____."

Meaning: _____

Client:

" _____."

Meaning: _____

" _____."

Meaning: _____

Breath

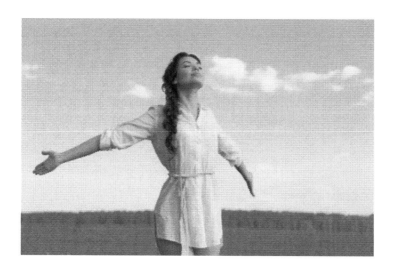

Breathing is one of the best things we can do for ourselves.

Breathe deep and bring the fresh oxygen into our lungs.

Exhale to let go of the toxins we don't want to hold onto.

Make ourselves comfortable with our own breathing.

It's free.

It's rejuvenating.

It helps you to be you.

How many times do we hold our breath when we are concentrating and we don't notice?

Breath is life enhancing so don't be afraid of it, get to know it!

Breath

Watch These To Learn More.

1. How Breathing Works by Nirvair Kaur

   http://ed.ted.com/lessons/how-breathing-works-nirvair-kaur

2. Breathing Lessons

   https://vimeo.com/35913315

3. Expanding The Movement Of The Breath

https://www.youtube.com/watch?v=WRYuzHmVaUU

An Awareness Through Movement® Feldenkrais Lesson

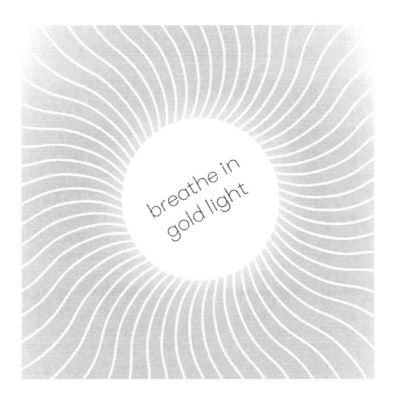

Bubbles

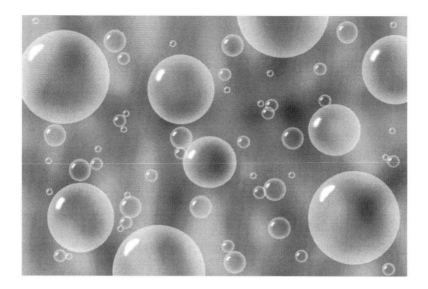

If you have a head injury or a memory problem it is a gift to the rest of the world. Truly, it is and you have a lot to teach others who are working with you if they are Doctors, Nurses, Therapists & Caregivers

You have information inside of your brain. With a trauma or accident, the retrieval of information has changed. It is often intimidating when a Doctor asks you how you are and then glosses over it because he or she doesn't have the time that you need to have the bubble of information come to you.

But remember, you are there to help them learn about brain injury.
You are there to ask the questions that will help you.

What To Do If You Are Flustered, Anxious or Embarrassed:

When someone asks you a question, ask them if they have the time to wait for your response because you have a head injury, and it takes longer to find and get the information out of you.

Either way they answer, you win because you were a teacher to help them learn about you and you kept your self-esteem. You don't need to be embarrassed because it takes you longer to find the information. Our world is fast and busy. No one has the time to smell the roses, but you ARE giving everyone the opportunity to stop for a few minutes and learn about you.

You may have a head injury, but you **DO** have a choice.
If you accept yourself now, you help people grow and become
more sensitive to people who have brain injuries and memory problems.

Calendars & Cues

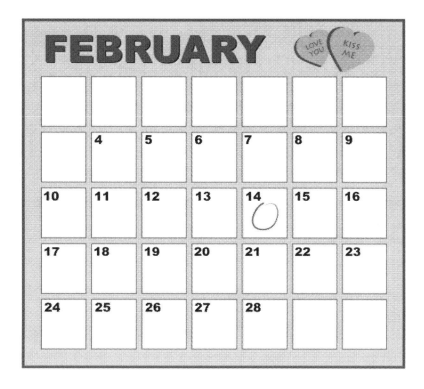

Lesson One

Put the important occasions on a large calendar somewhere the client has easy access to and is a simple place to cue him/her where to look.

Lesson Two

A big calendar that you can buy from an office supply store is an easy way for someone to know what they are involved in and that their life matters. Have the caregiver or the client record 1-3 things that happened to them on a daily basis.

Lesson Three

Have the caregiver or the client point to a day or choose a day for the client to see and read what he did that day. This is a strengthening memory exercise if this is done on a regular basis.

Calendars & Cues

This is an easy way for a client to see what he has done during the day, the week, the month, past months.

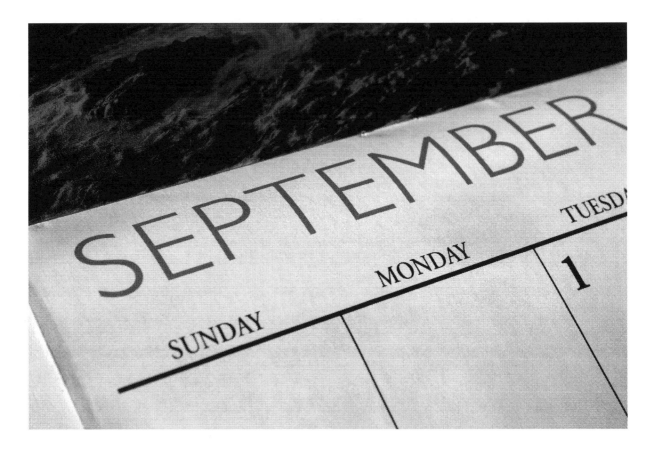

Celebration

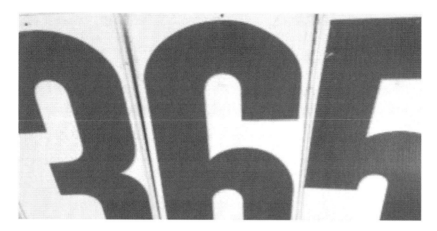

Celebrate You!

You are alive and that is a good thing.

Lesson One:

Find ways for you and your Caregiver to celebrate the day.

_____

_____

_____

_____

Lesson Two:

Find ways for you and your Client to celebrate the day.

_____

_____

_____

_____

Celebration

Lesson Three:

Find ways to celebrate the day together.

1._____

2._____

3._____

4._____

5._____

6._____

7._____

8._____

9._____

10._____

11._____

12._____

13._____

14._____

15._____

16._____

17._____

18._____

19._____

20._____

Certificate of Amazingness and Approval

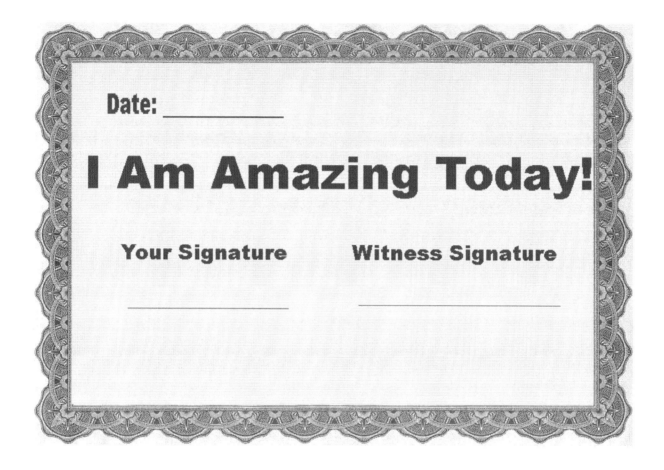

Lesson One:

Print out the full sized version on the back and make sure The Client and

The Caregiver give these awards out to each other as often as possible.

Caregiver & Client

Date: _____

I Am Amazing Today!

Your Signature   Witness Signature

_____   _____

Date: _____

I Am Amazing Today!

Your Signature   Witness Signature

_____   _____

Comfort Zone

It's where our basic needs are met and we feel satisfaction. We feel good about life.

It's difficult to get out of our comfort zone but it's also important to know what is our comfort zone.

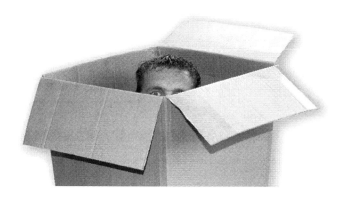

Lesson One:

What is my comfort zone?

Client

1._____

2._____

3._____

4._____

Comfort Zone

Caregiver

1._____

2._____

3._____

4._____

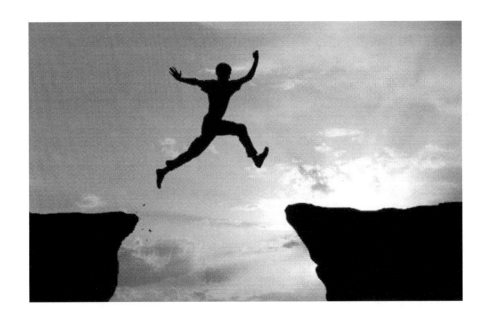

Comfort Zone

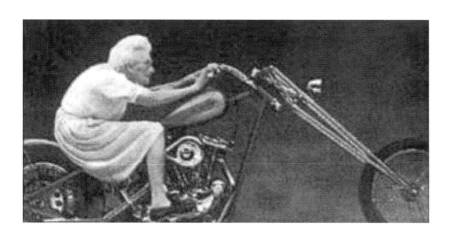

Lesson Two:

How can I expand my comfort zone?

Even though it seems like a huge leap for me and it makes me feel awkward.

Caregiver

1._____

2._____

3._____

4._____

Comfort Zone

Client

1._____

2._____

3._____

4._____

Comfort Zone

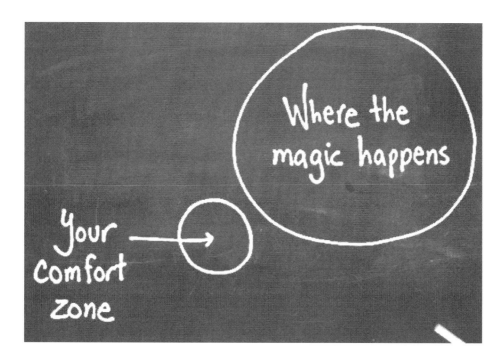

The good news is you expand your comfort zone a little bit at a time.

Lesson Three:

What are you finding out about this?

Client

1._____

2._____

3._____

4._____

Comfort Zone

Caregiver

1._____

2._____

3._____

4._____

Comfort Zone

Brené Brown is an American scholar, author, and public speaker, who is currently a research professor at the University of Houston Graduate College of Social Work. She studies and has written books on the topics of vulnerability, courage, authenticity and shame. She believes that the comfort zone is "where our uncertainty, scarcity and vulnerability are minimized - where we believe we'll have access to enough love, food, talent, time, admiration. Where we feel we have some control."

Brené Brown is a positive force for accepting who we are and having the courage to be who we are. Brené Brown studies vulnerability, courage, authenticity, and shame.

Her website is:

http://brenebrown.com

https://www.ted.com/talks/brene_brown_listening_to_shame

https://www.ted.com/talks/brene_brown_on_vulnerability?language=en

Books she has written:

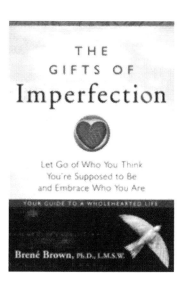
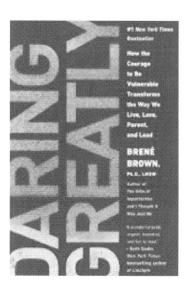
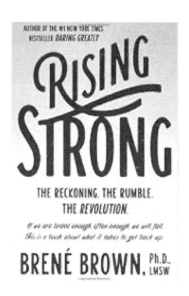

Lesson Four: How are you getting out of your comfort zone?

Caregiver:

_____

_____

_____

Client:

_____

_____

_____

Checklists For Daily Activities

Keep it simple so you can get this items done and you feel great.

Checklist for 3

Client   **Caregiver**

1._____   1._____

2._____   2._____

3._____   3._____

Yay!

Checklists For Daily Activities

Keep it simple so you can get this items done and you feel great.

Checklist for 5

Client   **Caregiver**

1._____   1._____

2._____   2._____

3._____   3._____

4._____   **4.**_____

5._____   5._____

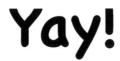

Checklists For Daily Activities

Keep it simple so you can get this items done and you feel great.

Checklist for 7

Client	**Caregiver**
1._____	1._____
2._____	2._____
3._____	3._____
4._____	**4.**_____
5._____	5._____
6._____	**6.**_____
7._____	7._____

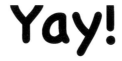

Checklists For Daily Activities

Keep it simple so you can get this items done and you feel great.

Checklist for 10

Client   **Caregiver**

1._____   1._____

2._____   2._____

3._____   3._____

4._____   **4.**_____

5._____   5._____

6._____   **6.**_____

7._____   7._____

8._____   8._____

9._____   **9.**_____

10._____   10._____

Yay!

Color

Color makes our life vivid and vibrant. There are many thoughts, books and resources that investigate the healing sources of color.

Lesson One:

Answer these questions and turn to the other side to see what the meanings of these colors are that I've gathered from

http://www.empower-yourself-with-color-psychology.com/meaning-of-colors.html

This is just some of the information presented on their website. You can go to this website for further information. It's a great way to understand colors and how they affect you. Investigate further with doing searches on color on the web.

Color Choices for this exercise

Red, Orange, Yellow, Green, Blue, Indigo, Purple, Turquoise, Pink, Magenta,

Brown, Gray, Silver, Gold, White, Black

	Client	Caregiver
What is your favorite color?	_____	_____
What color is your heart today?	_____	_____
What color is your mind today?	_____	_____
What color is your body today?	_____	_____
What color is your emotion today?	_____	_____
What color are your possibilities today?	_____	_____

Read your information to one another because it's a way to have conversation and learn from each other.

Color

The information was taken from

http://www.empower-yourself-with-color-psychology.com/meaning-of-colors.html

1. Red

This color is a warm and positive color associated with our most physical needs and our will to survive. It exudes a strong and powerful masculine energy. Red is energizing. It excites the emotions and motivates us to take action. It signifies a pioneering spirit and leadership qualities, promoting ambition and determination. It is also strong-willed and can give confidence to those who are shy or lacking in will power. Being the color of physical movement, the color red awakens our physical life force.

2. Orange

The color orange radiates warmth and happiness, combining the physical energy and stimulation of red with the cheerfulness of yellow. Orange relates to 'gut reaction' or our gut instincts, as opposed to the physical reaction of red or the mental reaction of yellow. Orange offers emotional strength in difficult times. It helps us to bounce back from disappointments and despair, assisting in recovery from grief.

3. Yellow

This color relates to acquired knowledge. It is the color which resonates with the left or logic side of the brain stimulating our mental faculties and creating mental agility and perception. Being the lightest hue of the spectrum. Yellow is the best color to create enthusiasm for life and can awaken greater confidence and optimism. The color yellow loves a challenge, particularly a mental challenge.

4. Green

This is the color of balance and harmony. From a color psychology perspective, it is the great balancer of the heart and the emotions, creating equilibrium between the head and the heart. From a meaning of colors perspective, green is also the color of growth, the color of spring, of renewal and rebirth. It renews and restores depleted energy. It is the sanctuary away from the stresses of modern living, restoring us back to a sense of well being. This is why there is so much of this relaxing color on the earth, and why we need to keep it that way. Green is an emotionally positive color, giving us the ability to love and nurture ourselves and others unconditionally. A natural peacemaker, it must avoid the tendency to become a martyr.

Color

5. Blue

This color is one of trust, honesty and loyalty. It is sincere, reserved and quiet, and doesn't like to make a fuss or draw attention. It hates confrontation, and likes to do things in its own way. Blue is reliable and responsible. This color exhibits an inner security and confidence. You can rely on it to take control and do the right thing in difficult times. It has a need for order and direction in its life, including its living and work spaces. This is a color that seeks peace and tranquility above everything else, promoting both physical and mental relaxation. It reduces stress, creating a sense of calmness, relaxation and order.

6. Indigo

The color indigo is the color of intuition and perception and is helpful in opening the third eye. It promotes deep concentration during times of introspection and meditation, helping you achieve deeper levels of consciousness. It relies on intuition rather than gut feeling. Indigo is a deep midnight blue. It is a combination of deep blue and violet and holds the attributes of both these colors. Service to humanity is one of the strengths of the color indigo. Powerful and dignified, indigo conveys integrity and deep sincerity.

7. Purple

This color relates to the imagination and spirituality. It stimulates the imagination and inspires high ideals. It is an introspective color, allowing us to get in touch with our deeper thoughts. The difference between violet and purple is that violet appears in the visible light spectrum, or rainbow, whereas purple is simply a mix of red and blue. Violet has the highest vibration in the visible spectrum. While the violet is not quite as intense as purple, its essence is similar.,Generally the names are interchangeable and the meaning of the colors is similar. Both contain the energy and strength of red with the spirituality and integrity of blue. This is the union of body and soul creating a balance between our physical and our spiritual energies.

8. Turquoise

The meaning of the color turquoise is open communication and clarity of thought. Turquoise helps to open the lines of communication between the heart and the spoken word. It presents as a friendly and happy color enjoying life. Turquoise controls and heals the emotions creating emotional balance and stability. This is a color that recharges our spirits during times of mental stress and tiredness, alleviating feelings of loneliness. You only have to focus on the color turquoise, whether on a wall or clothing and you feel instant calm and gentle invigoration, ready to face the world again!

Color

9. Pink

The meaning of the color pink is unconditional love and nurturing. This color represents compassion, nurturing and love. It relates to unconditional love and understanding, and the giving and receiving of nurturing. Pink is feminine and romantic, affectionate and intimate, thoughtful and caring. It tones down the physical passion of red replacing it with a gentle loving energy. Pink is intuitive and insightful, showing tenderness and kindness with its empathy and sensitivity.

10. Magenta

The color magenta is one of universal harmony and emotional balance. It is spiritual yet practical, encouraging common sense and a balanced outlook on life. This is a color that helps to create harmony and balance in every aspect of life; physically, mentally, emotionally and spiritually. Magenta influences our whole personal and spiritual development. It strengthens our intuition and psychic ability while assisting us to rise above the everyday dramas of our daily life to experience a greater level of awareness and knowledge.

11. Brown

This is the color of security, protection and material wealth. It is a serious, down-to- earth color signifying stability, structure and support. Relating to the protection and support of the family unit, with a keen sense of duty and responsibility, brown takes its obligations seriously. It encourages a strong need for security and a sense of belonging, with family and friends being of utmost importance. The color brown relates to quality in everything - a comfortable home, the best food and drink and loyal companionship. It is a color of physical comfort, simplicity and quality.

12. Gray

The color gray is the color of detachment,indecision and compromise.unemotional color. It is detached, neutral, impartial and indecisive - the fence- sitter. It is the color of compromise - being neither black nor white, it is the transition between two non-colors. The closer gray gets to black, the more dramatic and mysterious it becomes.The closer it gets to silver or white, the more illuminating and lively it becomes. Being both motionless and emotionless, gray is solid and stable and creates a sense of calm and composure. It provides relief from a chaotic world. The color gray is subdued, quiet and reserved. It does not stimulate, energize, rejuvenate or excite.

Color

13. Silver

Silver is the color of illumination and reflection. It has a feminine energy; it is related to the moon and the ebb and flow of the tides - it is fluid, emotional, sensitive and mysterious. It is soothing, calming and purifying. From a color psychology viewpoint, it signals a time of reflection and a change of direction as it illuminates the way forward. It helps with the cleansing and releasing of mental, physical and emotional issues and blockages as it opens new doors and lights the way to the future. With its reflective and sensitive qualities silver inspires - intuition, clairvoyance and mental telepathy. It reflects back any energy given out, whether it is positive or negative.

14. Gold

It is the color of wealth, success, achievement, triumph and royalty. It is associated with abundance and prosperity, luxury and quality, prestige and sophistication, value and elegance, Gold in its physical state, by its very nature, denotes wealth and prestige in every country, culture and market in the world today - it is probably the most valuable and easily traded commodity available in the global market place. This color is linked to masculine energy and the power of the sun, compared to silver which is associated with feminine energy and the sensitivity of the moon. Gold is the color of the winner - first place medals are always in gold.

15. White

White is color at its most complete and pure, the color of perfection. The color meaning of white is purity, innocence, wholeness and completion. It is the color of new beginnings, wiping the slate clean, so to speak. While white isn't stimulating to the senses, it opens the way for the creation of anything the mind can conceive. White contains an equal balance of all the colors of the spectrum, representing both the positive and negative aspects of all colors. Its basic feature is equality, implying fairness and impartiality, neutrality and independence.

16. Black

The color black relates to the hidden, the secretive and the unknown, and as a result it creates an air of mystery. It keeps things bottled up inside, hidden from the world. This color gives protection from external emotional stress. It creates a barrier between itself and the outside world, providing comfort while protecting its emotions and feelings, and hiding its vulnerabilities,

Color

16. Black

insecurities and lack of self confidence. Black is the absorption of all color and the absence of light. Black hides, while white brings to light. What black covers, white uncovers. We all use black at various times to hide from the world around us in one way or another. Some of us use it to hide our weight; others among us use it to hide our feelings, our fears or our insecurities. Black means power and control, hanging on to information and things rather than giving out to others.

Read further about your color choices from this website where I got the basic information.

http://www.empower-yourself-with-color-psychology.com/meaning-of-colors.html

Lesson Two:	**Client**	**Caregiver**
Has your color choice changed?	Yes/No	Yes/No
	_____	_____

Lesson Three:

From the information you just read about colors, please name 3 colors you need in your life.

Client:
1._____

2._____

3._____

Caregiver:
1._____

2._____

3._____

Lesson Four:

Now bring those colors into your life with the clothes you wear and color cards around your environment so you can bring this color into your life to live it.

Communication

Communication is a two way street. Here are some questions you can ask to get the conversation going? Both take turn asking the questions. Both get practice being the speaker and the listener.

Conversation starters
Lesson One: Ask Questions to each other. Find out information.

1. If you could thank anyone either living or passed on, who would it be?

2. What do you want from life now?

3. Which food do you feel nourishes you?

4. If you were trapped in an elevator who would you want it to be with?

5. Who would make you feel the most uncomfortable if you were trapped in an elevator with them?

6. If you could write a book, what would the title be called and what would it be about?

7. What do you like the most about yourself?

8. What would you like to change about yourself?

9. Can you say to yourself that you love who you are?

10. Find a newspaper or go to your computer, smartphone, iPad and see what today's current event is anywhere in the world, our country, the state you live in and/or the city or your neighborhood.

11. If your house is on fire and you have to get out, what is the the one thing you'd grab and save?

12. Who do you love?

13. Who loves you?

14. What would you like your family and friends to remember about you when you pass on?

15. What does success mean to you?

Communication

Conversation starters

16. Name 5 successful experiences you have had in the past.

17. Name 5 successful experiences you have had NOW.

18. What DON'T people get about you?

19. Name 1-5 movies that make you laugh.

20. Name 1-5 movies that make you cry.

21. What do you remember most growing up as a young child?

22. What do you remember most growing up as a teenager?

23. Name 5 traits your father gave you .

24. Name 5 traits your mother gave you.

25. What are you most grateful for?

26. If you could bring back any historical figure who would you bring back and why?

27. Do you think men and women view love in the same way?

28. What does love mean for you?

29. What songs do you love to listen to over and over again?

30. What type of music is your favorite type of music to listen to?

31. Who is our President?

32. If you could learn any language what language would that be?

33. Can you tell me a joke?

34. What is your favorite thing to do?

35. Which animals would you like to have as pets?

36. What is your favorite meal for breakfast?

37. What is your favorite meal for lunch?

Communication

Conversation starters

38. What is your favorite meal for dinner?

39. What is your favorite snack?

40. If you could bring back someone you loved to be with them for 30 minutes, what would you say to them?

41. What is your craft? What do you have a knack for? What would you do over and over again even if you didn't get paid?

42. If you could change anything about yourself, what would it be?

43. What physical feature do you notice first in the opposite sex?

44. If you could live anywhere, where would you live and why?

45. What invention do you believe to be the greatest of all time?

46. What is a favorite book of yours?

47. Do you believe there is life other than on earth?

48. When was the happiest day of your life?

49. You can have as many happy days to remember as possible. Try to remember as many as you can.

50. Name the funniest thing that ever happened to you.

51. Name the place that you have traveled to that you have enjoyed the most and why?

52. If could travel anywhere, where would you travel to and why?

53. Movement is life so name the movement that best describes you. Walking, talking, running, smiling, hugging, driving, skiing, swimming, etc...

54. Do you have a favorite saying that helps you in life?

55. What is one of your favorite personal stories to tell?

Communication

Lesson Two: What are your top ten questions for finding information about each other?

1._____

2._____

3._____

4._____

5._____

6._____

7._____

8._____

9._____

10._____

Compassion

Lesson One: "You can train your brain to learn it". Read the article by Helen Weng to see if you are interested in learning this free 30 minute meditation on compassion.

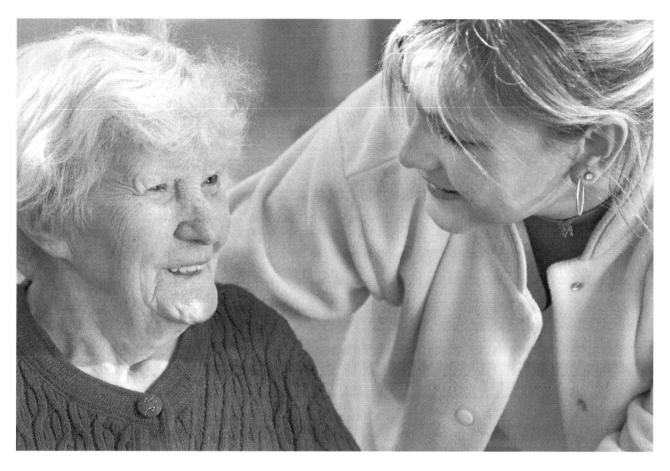

Learn more in this article written by Helen Weng

http://www.fastcoexist.com/3037045/want-to-train-your-brain-to-feel-more-compassion-heres-how

Helen Weng is a post-doctoral scholar at UCSF's Osher Center for Integrative Medicine where she studied 'mind-body interventions and relational functioning. She completed her work as a doctoral student in clinical psychology in 2014, conducting research at the University of Wisconsin-Madison's Center for Investigating Healthy Minds at the Waisman Center. Her research on compassion training was published in Psychological Science.

http://www.psychologicalscience.org/index.php/news/releases/compassion-training.html

Compassion

Lesson Two: This is where you sign up to receive a compassion training audio download. This would be a good thing for both the caregiver and the client to do together.

http://www.investigatinghealthyminds.org/compassion.html

Lesson Three: Are you listening to this compassion training audio on a regular basis.

Yes _____ No _____

Lesson Four: Write down what you are learning.

Caregiver:

_____

_____

_____

_____

Client:

_____

_____

_____

_____

Feelings

Feeling Feelings are important to acknowledge throughout the day for both the caregiver and client. Giving expression to your feelings helps to move through feelings and recognize they are always changing.

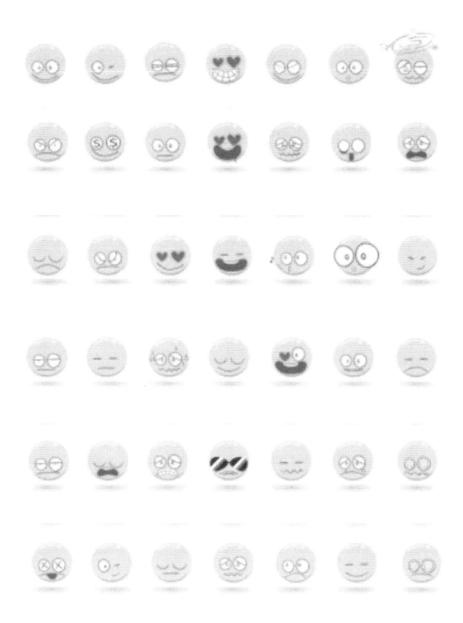

Knowing How You Feel Creates The Choices In Your Day

Feelings

Lesson One

Go thru each feeling and label it. Both the caregiver and client need to name the expression on the emoticon's face, so you have the same language when you are talking about these feelings.

Caregiver:

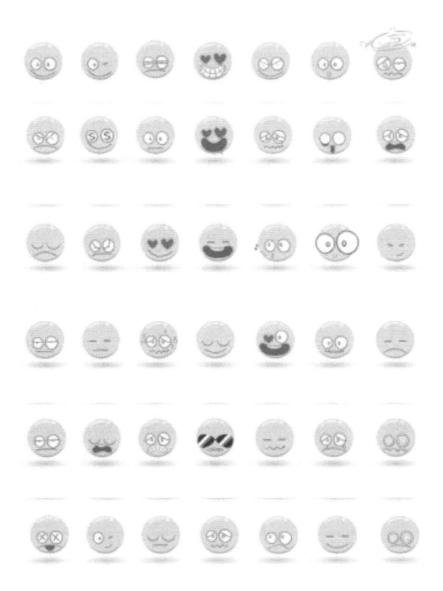

Knowing How You Feel Creates The Choices In Your Day

Feelings

Client:

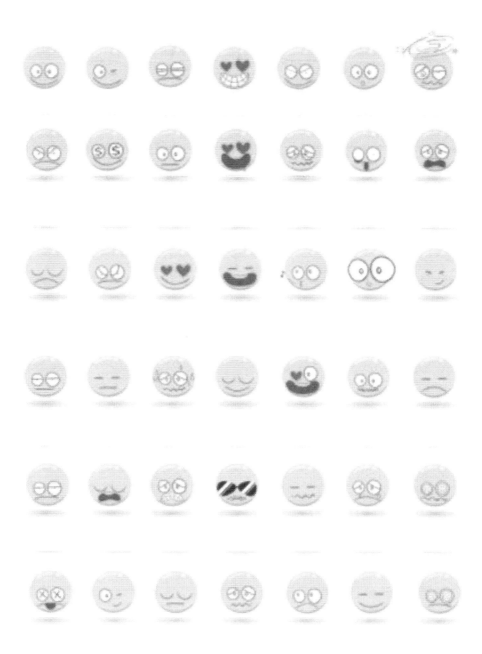

Knowing How You Feel Creates The Choices In Your Day

Feelings

Every four hours circle the feeling you are feeling and write it down here so you both can discuss what has happened throughout the day and evening.

A. Do your feelings stay the same or do they change?

B. If you had to give one feeling for the day what would it be? C. Negative feelings can be felt and diffused when named.

Joyful, happy, loving feelings can be pulled into the center of your heart and remembered by placing your hands on your heart, pausing for some moments and

feeling how good the love feels.

D. Give yourself or the client a blank piece of paper and color the emotion.

E. You can both give each other permission to leave the room and talk yourself through those feelings. Talk to the mirror or talk to the wall but not to any person who would be hurt by your words.

Client   **Caregiver**

_____   _____

_____   _____

_____   _____

_____   _____

This lesson is a great exercise to do ALL the time.

It helps the caregiver to avoid "burn out" and it helps the client to learn what he is feeling and how to control his expression of it in a better way.

The "Fight or Flight" Response

The "fight or flight" response is a behavioral pattern left over from when our survival depended upon us getting up and fleeing from a dangerous situation. Whenever we feel threatened, we go into an instinctual/automatic nervous system reaction from our sympathetic nervous system. No way could we be calm during this behavior pattern because we feel like our lives are in danger and so our body prepares to do battle with an unknown enemy. Our pupils start to dilate. The heart rate and blood pressure increases and our muscles get ready to spring into action for the run of their life. The blood vessels constrict and get thinner. Cold perspiration breaks out all over us, and we have thick, sticky and tacky saliva. Our digestive enzymes decrease, and so does the movement of food and the blood moves away from the gastrointestinal tract because we're not going to be stopping to eat. We think, feel and react like we are in danger. Our endocrine system is activated because we need all gears in place to get us out of danger.

This response consists of three parts. The first is a physical or verbal attack. The second part is a physical flight in which the person removes himself from the third part, and the third situation involves an emotional or psychological flight or withdrawal.

(Information Gotten from Neurophysiological Concepts in Human Behavior, The Tree of Learning) By Margot C. Heiniger and Shirley L. Randolph. The C.V. Mosby Company, 1981

Understanding where you and the caregiver are on this continuum and where you and the client are on this continuum is vital to recognize and explore.

The "Fight or Flight" Response

Lesson One:

Both of you spend some time talking about past situations you felt like a physical fight, verbal attack, physically removing yourself from the situation or emotionally removing yourself from the situation.

Lesson Two:

Both of you spend some time talking about immediate situations involving both of you that felt like a physical fight, verbal attack, physically removing yourself from the situation or emotionally removing yourself from the situation.

Lesson Three:

Name your stress triggers that put thou in a "fight or flight" response.

Caregiver   **Client**

1.   _____   _____

2.   _____   _____

3.   _____   _____

4.   _____   _____

5.   _____   _____

6.   _____   _____

7.   _____   _____

8.   _____   _____

9.   _____   _____

10. _____   _____

The "Fight or Flight" Response

Lesson Four:

Read the information aloud that is presented on this website.

http://www.thebodysoulconnection.com/EducationCenter/fight.html

Lesson Five:

Watch the video checklist of physical and emotional symptoms that accompany an overactive fight or flight response.

http://www.thebodysoulconnection.com/EducationCenter/fight.html

Lesson Six:

What are some good take away points from reading the information and watching the video.

Client	Caregiver
1._____	_____
2._____	_____
3._____	_____
4._____	_____
5._____	_____
6._____	_____
7._____	_____
8._____	_____
9._____	_____
10._____	_____

The "Fight or Flight" Response

Lesson Seven:
Develop each other's plan to minimize these "fight or flight" responses.

Plan From The Caregiver to The Client For Decreasing "Fight or Flight" Responses:

_____

_____

_____

_____

_____

_____

_____

_____

Plan From The Client to The Caregiver For Decreasing "Fight or Flight" Responses:

_____

_____

_____

_____

_____

_____

_____

_____

Focus

We are a world of distractions with noises, chit chatter and commercials trying to distract us from our thoughts about who we really are. Focusing is the first step in learning how to quiet the mind chatter from within yourself.

Lesson One:
Take one minute to focus on nothing or a picture or a word and notice what happens.

Caregiver Notices What   **Client Notices What**

_____   _____

Lesson Two:
Take two minutes to focus on nothing or a picture or a word and notice what happens.

Caregiver Notices What   **Client Notices What**

_____   _____

Lesson Three:
Take five minutes to focus on nothing or a picture or a word and notice what happens.

Caregiver Notices What   **Client Notices What**

_____   _____

Lesson Four:
Take ten minutes to focus on nothing or a picture or a word and notice what happens.

Caregiver Notices What   **Client Notices What**

_____   _____

Lesson Five:
Take fifteen minutes to focus on nothing or a picture or a word and notice what happens.

Caregiver Notices What   **Client Notices What**

_____   _____

Focus

Lesson Six:

See how long you can focus on this bullseye

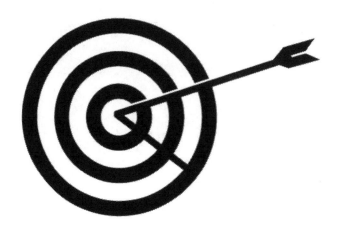

	Client	**Caregiver**
First Time	_____	_____
Second Time	_____	_____
Third Time	_____	_____
Fourth Time	_____	_____
Fifth Time	_____	_____
Sixth Time	_____	_____
Seventh Time	_____	_____
Eight Time	_____	_____
Ninth Time	_____	_____
Tenth Time	_____	_____

FORGIVENESS

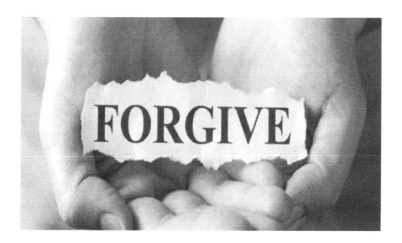

· It is a good practice to forgive those you know have done you wrong.
· It is a good practice forgive those you think have done you wrong.
It is a good practice to forgive those you have no idea you need to forgive.

Lesson One: In the silence of your heart and soul forgive who you would like to forgive.

Lesson Two: In the silence of your heart and soul forgive yourself

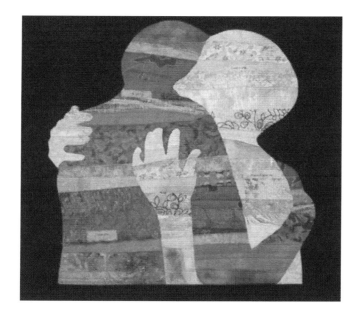

FORGIVENESS

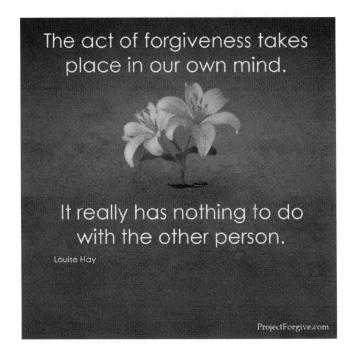

Lesson Three:http://projectforgive.com

Go there for inspiration, community and support

Going Fishing

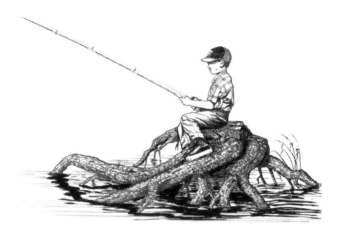

Chinese Proverb

Give a man a fish and you feed him for a day.
Teach a man to fish and you feed him for a lifetime.

This proverb, of course is for women and children as well.

Going Fishing

Lesson One:

What do you need to go fishing for the rest of your life?

Caregiver:

_____

_____

_____

_____

_____

_____

Going Fishing

Client:

_____

_____

_____

_____

_____

_____

Going Out in The Community

It just makes sense doesn't it to be a part of your community, doesn't it?

Community Centers

Churches

Local Parks

Stores you like to shop at

Going to the Post Office

Taking a ride on the bus

Going for a walk around your community

Taking classes

Support Groups

Exercise One:

How are you part of your community?

Client	**Caregiver**
_____	_____
_____	_____
_____	_____
_____	_____

Going Out in The Community

Lesson Two:

Plan to go out on a community outing together

What are the steps involved to go out in the community

Step 1 _____

Step 2 _____

Step 3 _____

Step 4 _____

Step 5 _____

Lesson Three:

Go out and work your plan.

Lesson Four:

How did it go? Would you do anything differently

_____

_____

_____

Lesson Five:

Make another plan to go out in the community and repeat as often as you can.

_____

_____

_____

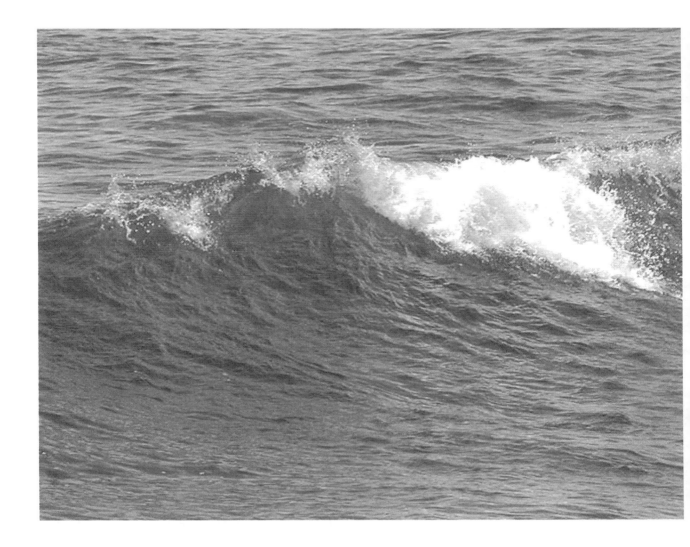

Healing

Healing who you are is about making yourself feel like you are okay within yourself, that you are feeling whole with all of yourself - your body, mind, emotions, energy, heart, spirit and soul.

Lesson One:

Ask yourself this question: Do you feel whole and healthy?

Caregiver: Yes _____   No _____

Why: 1._____

          2._____

          3._____

Client: Yes _____   No _____

Why: 1._____

          2._____

          3._____

Healing

Lesson Two:

Go to this blog: http://zenhabits.net/heal/ and and read this blog together.

Lesson Three: Write down the 6 steps to healing by Lissa Rankin

1._____

2._____

3._____

4._____

5._____

6._____

Lesson Four:

Go thru each step and check off if you believe this is possible within yourself.

Step One

Believe You Can Heal Yourself

Client: Yes_____   No_____

Caregiver: Yes_____   No_____

Step Two:

Find The Right Support.

Client: Yes_____   No_____

Caregiver: Yes_____   No_____

Step Three:

Listen To Your Body & Your Intuition

Client: Yes_____   No_____

Caregiver: Yes_____   No_____

Healing

Step Four:
Diagnose The Root Cause Of Your Disease

Client: Yes_____   No_____

Caregiver: Yes_____   No_____

Step Five:
Write The Prescription For Yourself

Client: Yes_____   No_____

Caregiver: Yes_____   No_____

Step Six:
Surrender Attachments To Outcomes

Client: Yes_____   No_____

Caregiver: Yes_____   No_____

Lesson Five:
Now talk with each other about this possibility.
Some questions to stimulate conversation:

1. Is this a possibility for you now?

2. What is your fear about moving forward in your life?

3. Can you name a time in your life when you knew this to be true?

4. Name people in your life who have healed themselves when they should not have.

5. Can you open up to the love and worth inside of your mind, body, heart, spirit and soul that can make this possible because you are yourself in oneness?

Healing

Lesson Six:

Read more about Lissa Rankin, MD on her website
www.LissaRankin.com.

She has free healing kits when you sign up for her blog.

She's written two books:

Mind Over Medicine: Scientific Proof That You Can Heal Yourself, offers all the scientific pr
skeptics will need in order to believe the mind really can heal the body. It also guides you
through a series of exercises to help you implement the 6 Steps To Healing Yourself so
you can make your body ripe for miracles.

The Fear Cure

And you can also go to this website as well for more information on her.
http://mindovermedicinebook.com

She is a wealth of information and it is worth your time to check out her website!

Inspiration

iPad, iPhone, Smartphone

1. Do you have one?   Yes_____   No_____

2. Do you know how to work one? Yes_____   No_____

3. Do you have a friend or a family member who can be a mentor in helping

    you learn more information.   Yes _____   No _____

    My Technology Mentor is: _____

Inspiration

4. There are many helpful applications besides

   calling someone, skyping, FaceTime, emailing and internet searching.

   There are applications to help you record messages to yourself.

   Take photos and videos.

   Daily reminders and organization.

   Voice recognition capabilities. *You talk and the application writes it down.*

Lesson One:

What would you like to use your device for?

Caregiver: **Client:**

_____   _____

_____   _____

_____   _____

Lesson Two:

Now that you know what you are looking for go to you local cell phone provider like Verizon, Sprint etc… and let their sales people sent their time and energy educating you about what their products can do for you.

Lesson Three:

Go to the closest Apple or Microsoft store and do the same thing. Let their sales people spend their time and energy talking to you about what they have.

Cues:

• 1:1 visits like these cost minimal amounts of money and you can go as often as you need to until your comfort level improves.

• Picking out an iPad, iPhone or Smartphone for just 1-2 things that will help you in your daily life is just fine.

Laughter

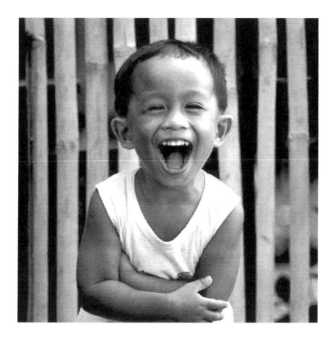

Laughter is a great way to release healthy, healing, happy energy throughout your body.

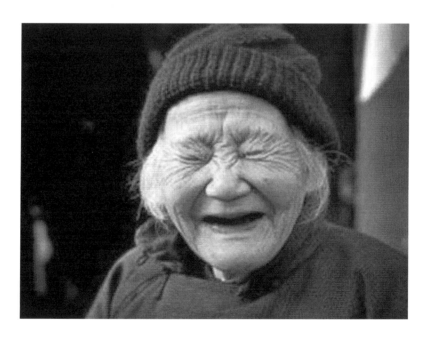

Laughter

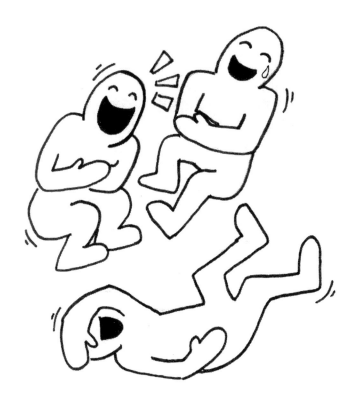

It's Healing and It's Contagious

Lesson One:

Tell The Joke

a. Knock- Knock

b. Who's there?

a. The Interrupting Cow.

b. Interrup

a. MOOOO!

Laughter

Lesson Two

Tell More Jokes

1. What did one ocean say to the other ocean?

Nothing, they just waved.

2. Why do hummingbirds hum?

Because they can't remember the words

Lesson Three

What makes you laugh? What makes you smile?
What T.V. Shows help you do this?

Client

Caregiver

_____ _____

_____ _____

_____ _____

_____ _____

_____ _____

_____ _____

_____ _____

_____ _____

_____ _____

_____ _____

Laughter

Lesson Four:
Find out more about the power of laughter through these websites.

Benefits of:

http://www.helpguide.org/articles/emotional-health/laughter-is-the-best-medicine.htm

http://www.webmd.com/balance/features/give-your-body-boost-with-laughter

http://articles.mercola.com/sites/articles/archive/2014/11/13/10-fascinating-facts-laughter.aspx

Laughter Places:

http://jokes.cc.com

http://www.rd.com/jokes/funny/

http://www.funology.com/jokes-and-riddles/

http://jokes4us.com/miscellaneousjokes/schooljokes/kidjokes.html

http://www.ahajokes.com

http://www.laughfactory.com/jokes

http://unijokes.com

http://www.punoftheday.com/cgi-bin/disppuns.pl?ord=F

Living With A Head Injury

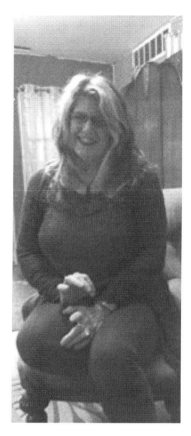

I've known Leah Parker for over twenty-five years. I knew her before her head injury and I know her after her head injury. She's a beautiful woman at sixty something. Yet, she's had to struggle to overcome her head injury. She's also had to accept that she has memory problems.

She lives in Santa Barbara now but comes back to Seattle to "catch up" with old friends and see clients who won't give her up. She's a gifted healer in the areas of massage, astrology, hypnotherapy and star essences. She came to teach The Star Essences Certification Course to Elthea and me in May, 2015. It was a magical sunny weekend with these wonderful women in my Yurt.

The class lasted ten hours for two days and an initial evening a few days before for three hours. It was a detailed class and it took a great deal of energy to learn. I was tired. Elthea was tired. Leah was tired because she had to compensate for her memory issues. She bounced back after she gave herself some time to rest and sleep.

The Key: Rest and Sleep

The office staff at Star Essences color codes stickies to help Leah with the follow thru of steps in the workshop training. This process helps Leah with the basics of what she needs to do one step at a time from start to finish. This structure gives her the confidence with organizational needs.

I thought she was a wonderful teacher and I did not notice any "slip-ups" in the course. She laughed and said she covers it up well. I told her she's improved from two years prior when I took another weekend course with her. **Leah's a living example of neuroplasticity because she's unfolding her brain with possibilities and connecting her memory dots with what she loves to do and is engaged.**

Living With A Head Injury - Leah Parker

1. **Misconception about a head injury.** You're not as smart anymore and that's not the way it is. You're still you and you're still in you, you just have to get it out. It's the accessing and getting "you" out which is challenging.

2. **Many Dimensions to Head Injury**
Figure out how to get organized, even if you need a professional organizer to do this so you can accomplish your tasks this is okay. It is a good investment to get the executive help, assistance and organization you need for you, your home and your life.

3. **What I notice about myself** I feel scattered in terms of what's my order, executive function & motivation.

4. **What Helps?**
Assignment Sheets for sequencing and rhythm.
Post Its.
Focus helps me to get back into myself.
Doing something over and over.
DO what feeds and nourishes YOU.
Learn a little dance that balances my left and right side with movement.
Exercises with my body.
Crying when I feel "spent".
Walk outside when I feel "spent".
Have someone give me assignments to do. One at a time.
Find support at going to meetings for brain injury.
Give my brain a cooling rest by clocking myself out after 45 minutes or when my brain gets tired.
Star Flower Essences to increase frequency, clarity & initiative - Alchemy Action
https://www.staressence.com

Living With A Head Injury

Lesson One:

What are your 3 "go to's" for living with a head injury.

Client

1._____

2._____

3._____

What are your 3 "go to's" for dealing effectively and successfully with someone who has a head injury.

Caregiver

1._____

2._____

3._____

Lesson Two:

Name three things you can do that Leah does to help her life.

1._____

2._____

3._____

What do I do that I love that can connect me to my memory dots?

Caregiver:

_____

_____

_____

_____

_____

_____

Client:

_____

_____

_____

_____

_____

_____

LUMOSITY

lumosity.com- Lumosity Brain Games

This is a website that was designed by neuroscientists to challenge your brain with games to exercise memory and attention with customized, personalized brain training programs for you. This is an excellent and wonderful website!

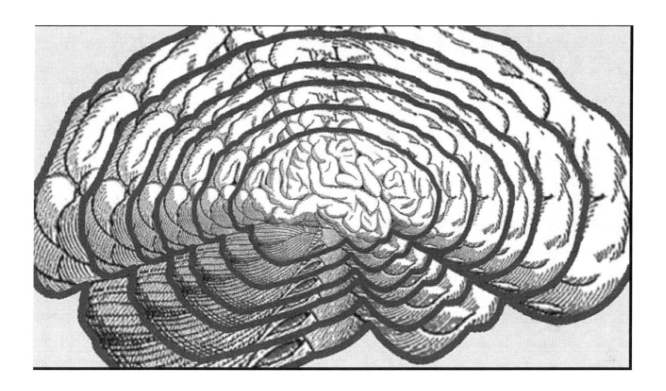

lumosity.com- Lumosity Brain Games

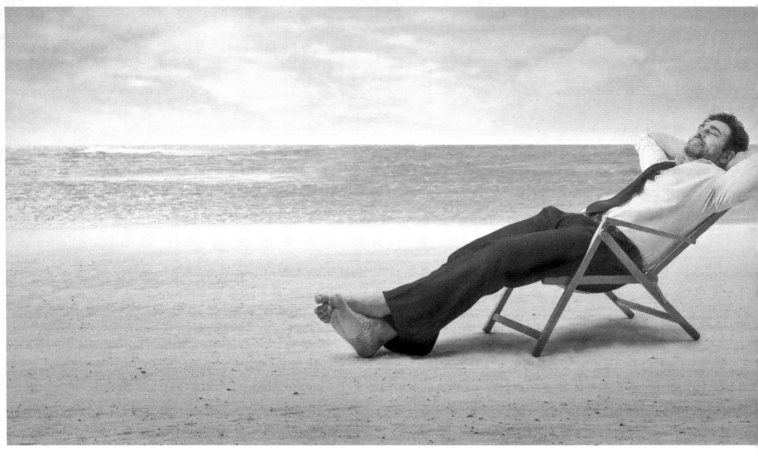

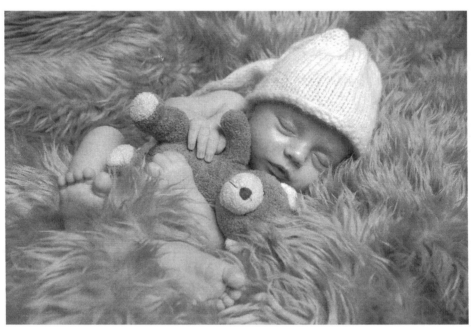

Make Yourself Comfortable

Lesson One: Right now I'd like you to make yourself comfortable. Do whatever it takes to try to get to that special place so we can see how you got there and then I want you to make note of the following:

Client:

Can you make yourself comfortable on your own?   Yes _____ No _____

Do you need someone else to make you comfortable? Yes _____ No_____

Do you need something else to make you comfortable Yes _____ No_____

What helps you to be comfortable?

_____,_____,_____,_____

Can you be comfortable anywhere?   Yes _____ No_____

Where are your best comfort environments?

_____

_____

_____

Does your clothing have something to do with your comfort?   Yes _____No_____

What clothing do you most prefer to be comfortable in?

_____

_____

_____

Are there times of the day and evening that are easier for you? Yes _____ No_____

If so, describe the times of the day that best work with your comfort level.

_____,_____ ._____

Describe what it means to you to be comfortable.

_____

_____

_____

_____

Make Yourself Comfortable

Lesson One: Right now I'd like you to make yourself comfortable. Do whatever it takes to try to get to that special place so we can see how you got there and then I want you to make note of the following:

Caregiver:

Can you make yourself comfortable on your own?   Yes _____ No _____

Do you need someone else to make you comfortable? Yes _____ No_____

Do you need something else to make you comfortable Yes _____ No_____

What helps you to be comfortable?

_____,_____,_____,_____

Can you be comfortable anywhere?   Yes _____ No_____

Where are your best comfort environments?

_____

_____

_____

Does your clothing have something to do with your comfort?   Yes _____No_____

What clothing do you most prefer to be comfortable in?

_____

_____

_____

Are there times of the day and evening that are easier for you?   Yes _____ No_____

If so, describe the times of the day that best work with your comfort level.

_____,_____._____

Describe what it means to you to be comfortable.

_____

_____

_____

_____

Make Yourself Comfortable

When you are comfortable and relaxed, it means your "fight or flight" response to life is switched off. You are not in survival mode but in a curious mode where you are willing to explore yourself and the environment with greater possibilities than when you are "shut down" in survival mode.

There's really only two approaches to life:

1). "Fight or flight" and it involves fear and reinforcing fear. SURVIVAL!

This involves your sympathetic nervous system and it's like revving a race car getting ready to take off. All systems go. The problem is when your system is revving up all the time, eventually the systems in your body break down because there has been "no" start or "end" to this race.

2). Comfort is all about being comfortable in your skin and it is about BEING CALM!

This involves the parasympathetic nervous system. Typically, this is the system we use to get a good night's rest or what gets activated in meditation and healing states of consciousness. This is the calming place of who we are. Interestingly enough, we can make ourselves more comfortable by noticing our breathing and taking the time to breathe deeply and making sure we get a good night's rest.

The Feldenkrais Method® with Functional Integration® and Awareness Through Movement® can help you with your own comfort. The four core principles of this method include the following:

1. Ease of movement.
2. The absence of resistance.
3. The presence of reversibility.
4. Comfortable breathing.

In Moshe Feldenkrais's book, The Potent Self, he indicates that "in good action, the sensation of effort is absent, no matter what the actual expenditure of energy is. It suffices to observe a good judo man, an expert weight-lifter, a figure-skating champion, a first-class acrobat, a great diva, an Arabian horseman -- in fact anybody who has learned to perform correctly mental or bodily actions -- in order to convince oneself that the sensation of effort is the subjective feeling of wasted movement."

Make Yourself Comfortable

"Furthermore, the sensation of resistance is produced when the muscles of the body prepare themselves to achieve a certain act, but do so in conflict with the rest of the self. We often try to remedy this situation by using what we call "will power." But "only immature people need will effort to act," says Feldenkrais."The mature person clears up all the irrelevant motivations and uses interest, necessity, and skill unhindered by unrecognized emotional urges."

The recognition of resistance is of utmost importance, because in ignoring it we will continue to act against ourselves, we will not be able to get rid of it, and when we see other people succeeding where we continue to fail, we will label ourselves with some kind of deficiency and turn away from the activity all together.

Reversibility means the capability to discontinue or reverse an act without effort, and without any change in attitude. This does of course take into consideration reflex actions or inertia. "The importance of reversibility," explains Feldenkrais, "is that it is possible only when there is fine control of excitation and inhibition , and a normal ebb and flow between the parasympathetic and the sympathetic. The test of reversibility holds good for all human activity, whether it is viewed from the physical or the emotional standpoint."

Lastly, comfortable breathing is desirable. Many people hold their breath constantly. Their body image propels them to continuously rearrange their throat, their chest, and their abdomen before they even speak. "In some the disturbance is so manifest," indicates Feldenkrais, " that the chest is fixed in the position of inspiration or expiration continuously. This upsets the normal ventilation, and has profound effects on the acid-base balance of the blood."

Observe a good judo man, an expert weight-lifter, a figure-skating champion, a first-class acrobat, a great diva, an Arabian horseman -- in fact anybody who has learned to perform correctly mental or bodily actions -- in order to convince oneself that the sensation of effort is the subjective feeling of wasted movement." Furthermore, the sensation of resistance is produced when the muscles of the body prepare themselves to achieve a certain act, but do so in conflict with the rest of the self. We often try to remedy this situation by using what we call "will power." But "only immature people need will effort to act," says Feldenkrais."The mature person clears up all the irrelevant motivations and uses interest, necessity, and skill unhindered by unrecognized emotional urges."

Make Yourself Comfortable

The recognition of resistance is of utmost importance, because in ignoring it we will continue to act against ourselves, we will not be able to get rid of it, and when we see other people succeeding where we continue to fail, we will label ourselves with some kind of deficiency and turn away from the activity all together. Reversibility means the capability to discontinue or reverse an act without effort, and without any change in attitude. This does of course take into consideration reflex actions or inertia. "The importance of reversibility," explains Feldenkrais, "is that it is possible only when there is fine control of excitation and inhibition , and a normal ebb and flow between the parasympathetic and the sympathetic. The test of reversibility holds good for all human activity, whether it is viewed from the physical or the emotional standpoint." Lastly, comfortable breathing is desirable. Many people hold their breath constantly. Their body image propels them to continuously rearrange their throat, their chest, and their abdomen before they even speak. a "In some the disturbance is so manifest," indicates Feldenkrais, " that the chest is fixed in the position of inspiration or expiration continuously. This upsets the normal ventilation, and has profound effects on the acid-base balance of the blood."

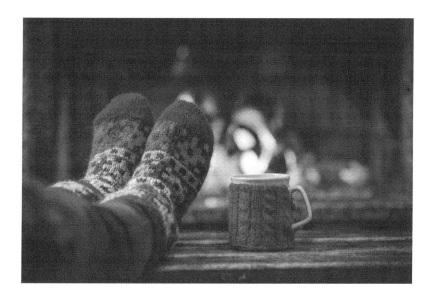

So 2 great take away points about comfort from Feldenkrais is this:

#1.   If you had to hold a position for eternity. How would you organize yourself so you could do this gently, effortlessly and elegantly.

#2.   Change your thought and your movement can become more comfortable.
Change your movement and your thoughts can become more comfortable.

Make Me Comfortable List

Client:

1._____

2._____

3._____

4._____

5._____

6._____

7._____

8._____

9._____

10._____

Caregiver:

1._____

2._____

3._____

4._____

5._____

6._____

7._____

8._____

9._____

10._____

Meditation

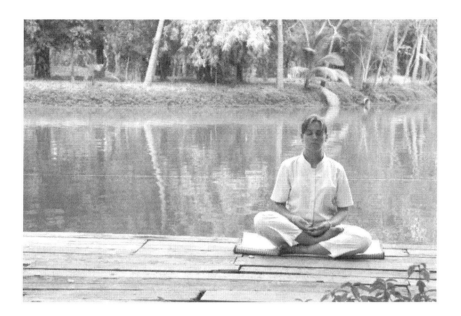

Meditation is applied focus repeating over and over again a word, a phrase, a sound or a chant. This calms the excessive mind chatter, negative talk or self-criticism that seems to happen when we are not mindful nor in our heart. It seems the mind loves to create havoc in our world and seems to think that it is the center of the universe. But, it is not. This is a hard lesson for the mind to learn that it is not all the center of the universe. So if we calm the mind then we have the possibility to know the much bigger world inside of us. There are so many ways to do a meditation, from sitting to walking, to using sounds that you can make it work according to who you are.

Meditation

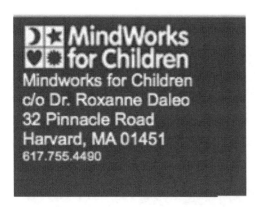

Mindworks for Children
c/o Dr. Roxanne Daleo
32 Pinnacle Road
Harvard, MA 01451
617.755.4490

Lesson One:
Dr. Roxanne Daleo
From Relax, Energize, Discover by Dr. Roxanne Dale
Mindworks™ 1988
Cambridge, MA

Your breath is a healing massage to let go of tension.
Let go.
Find a comfortable position so your body feels settled in one place. Uncross legs and arms.

Feet flat on floor. Back straight.
Allow your energy to flow freely. Throughout your body.
Breathe naturally and evenly.
Attention.
Breath
Center of your body just below your navel.
Breathe like a stream of fresh, clear water flow into your toes and feet.
Flow of relaxation circulating in toes and feet.
Sink down with every out breath- a let go into relaxation.
Automatically learn how to relax .
Let thoughts come and go like clouds.
Send flow of relaxation to calves
Like a clear of fresh stream of water.
Into your knees
Into your thighs
Into you abdomen
Flow into your chest and your back
Let your body sink down
Muscles are relaxed.
And your body is warm
Relaxation if moving and soothing throughout your body.
Your neck and your shoulders
Allow gravity to pull your shoulders down into the most relaxed position.
Upper arms, forearms, hands and out through your fingers
Muscles are relaxed
Breathe into your face
Muscles around your eyes and your forehead – the stress is draining out
Walking into a forest. Smell the freshness of the forest and the cool forest rain.

Meditation

Lesson Two:
Dr. Roxanne Daleo

A beautiful natural spring.
Warmed by the rays of the sun
Streaming down on it.
Dip into the warm. It's warm and inviting.
Sit into int, it goes up to your shoulders
Allow soothing warmth of the water as it circles around you like a gentle massage as you rest.

You breathe slowly and gently.
Muscles are relaxing.
Water is whirling and swirling around you and you are letting go of any tightness, any pain.

Warmth of water and movement of the water is soothing.

Can return anytime with breath.
Breathe in energy with exhale.
Allow the energy to flow more deeply, deeper and deeper into relaxation.
Return calm and refreshed.
Stretch your body.

More Information on Dr. Roxanne Daleo can be found on these websites.

http://www.mindworksforchildren.com

http://www.drroxannedaleo.com/?page_id=30

https://www.youtube.com/watch?v=0Pw8GKkMRYQ

Meditation

Lesson Three:

Go to these websites and explore a meditation that you would like to use.

https://www.psychologytoday.com/basics/meditation

http://www.meditationoasis.com/how-to-meditate/simple-meditations/

http://tinybuddha.com/blog/8-ways-to-make-meditation-easy-and-fun/

Client:

What Meditation are you going to start out with?

Remember, you can go to a youtube to have someone talk you through it.
Write down the meditation or put the website so you can remember where you need to go.

_____

_____

_____

_____

Caregiver:

What Meditation are you going to start out with?
Remember, you can go to a youtube to have someone talk you through it. Write down the meditation or put the website so you can remember where you need to go.

_____

_____

_____

_____

Memory - Brain, Gut, Muscle and Heart

1. Our heart remembers the most important stories about who we are.

2. Our brain is important because it helps us with our intuitive and logical sides.

3. The body and the brain help us with alertness and awareness.

4. Our heart, is where we feel our feelings and emotions.
   Feeling our feelings is what moves everything.
   Feeling our feelings allows us to feel the buoyancy of how we float (like the boat at the dock).
   Feeling our feelings moves us.
   If you pay attention to your feelings, you'll see your feelings change quite a bit.
   If we understand this we can let our feelings go once we have felt them.
   We don't have to be so bound up with repressed feelings.
   Feel feelings and let them go.

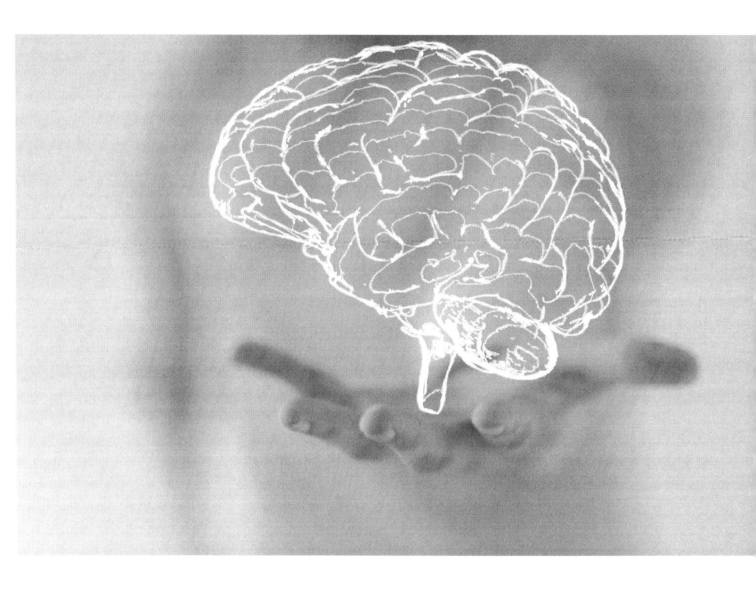

Memory Boards

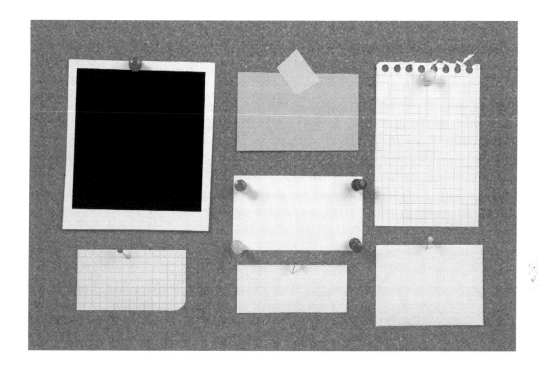

Buy some cork board, push pins or velcro.

Stick up your favorite words, pictures, quotes, thoughts, songs and music.

Whatever you want to remember.

What do you want to remember?

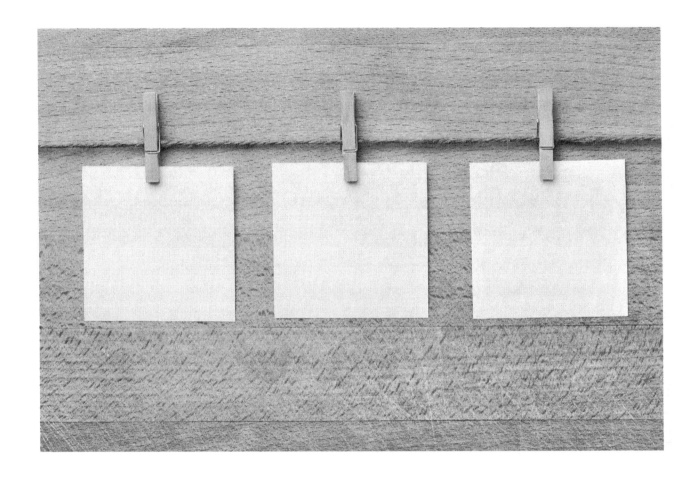

Movement

Our movement is made up of a combination of immature, mature and highly evolved movement patterns and motor plans. s

DO IT!

Activities and individual stress levels, personal habits and belief systems that affect the quality of our movement. Movement patterns also reflect the level of developmental integration for the coordinated activities of the mouth, tongue, eyes, lungs, pelvis, hips, legs, arms, feet & hand patterns.

Explore Your Movement

**Circular Movements are more natural.
They're in alignment to how our body moves.
Think circles with our different body parts.**

Eyes	Blinking. Opening. Closing. Together. Individually. Move from side to side. Up and Down. In a Circle. Then the opposite circle. Stare at yourself in the mirror
Ears	Head, Neck and Tongue. Move them around.
Mouth	Smiles,Frowns, Pouting, Puckering
Shoulders	Arms, Elbows
Hands	Holding them, Handshake, Patty Cake, Hold a bowl, Use a rolling pin
Thumb & Fingers	Touch
Breathing	
Back	Stomach & Pelvic Muscles
Legs	Feet. Toes. Walk. Talk

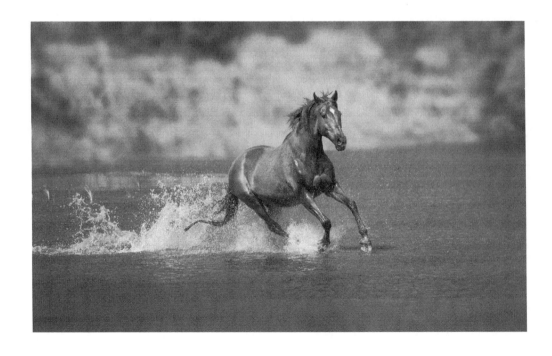

Music, Songs, Sing, Sound, Hum & Chant

Find the balance.

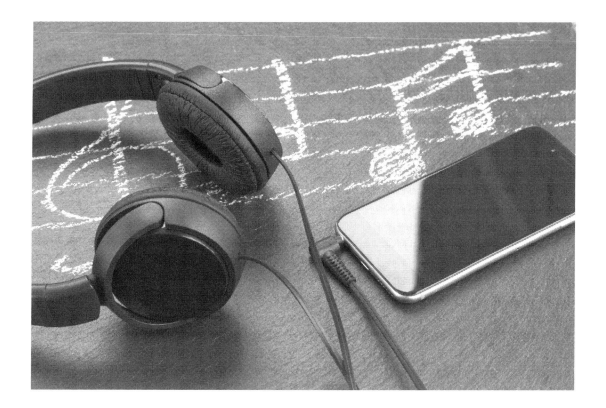

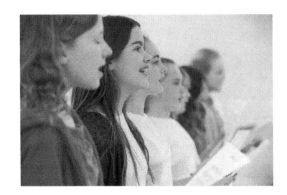

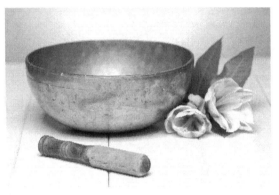

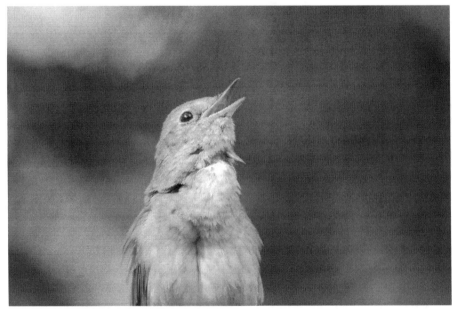

Nourish

What Nourishes You?

Client:

_____

_____

_____

_____

_____

_____

_____

_____

_____

_____

_____

_____

_____

_____

_____

_____

_____

_____

_____

_____

What Nourishes You?

Caregiver:

_____

_____

_____

_____

_____

_____

_____

_____

_____

_____

_____

_____

_____

_____

_____

_____

_____

_____

Novelty

Do things in a different way.

Try something different.

Surprise yourself.

Client
What You Did Differently   **How did you feel?**

_____   _____

_____   _____

_____   _____

_____   _____

_____   _____

_____   _____

_____   _____

_____   _____

_____   _____

_____   _____

_____   _____

_____   _____

_____   _____

Novelty

Do things in a different way.

Try something different.

Surprise yourself.

Caregiver:
What You Did Differently   **How did you feel?**

_____   _____

_____   _____

_____   _____

_____   _____

_____   _____

_____   _____

_____   _____

_____   _____

_____   _____

_____   _____

_____   _____

_____   _____

_____   _____

_____   _____

Organization and Simplifying

Less is better.

Declutter.

Get rid of the piles.

Clean out your closet.

Keep your life environment simple so you enjoy it.

What We Have Decluttered, Gotten Rid Of, Organized and Simplified.

Caregiver   **Client**

_____   _____

_____   _____

_____   _____

_____   _____

_____   _____

_____   _____

_____   _____

_____   _____

_____   _____

_____   _____

_____   _____

_____   _____

_____   _____

Less is better.

Declutter.

Get rid of the piles.

Clean out your closet.

Keep your life environment simple so you enjoy it.

What We Have Decluttered, gotten rid of, organized and simplified

Caregiver   **Client**

_____   _____

_____   _____

_____   _____

_____   _____

_____   _____

_____   _____

_____   _____

_____   _____

_____   _____

_____   _____

_____   _____

_____   _____

_____   _____

_____   _____

Our Bios

Regularly write out a one paragraph about who you are and put it on the refrigerator or the bulletin board or in a notebook. See how it changes.

Caregiver's Bio:

_____

_____

_____

_____

Client's Bio:

_____

_____

_____

_____

Caregiver's Bio:

_____

_____

_____

_____

Client's Bio:

_____

_____

_____

_____

Caregiver's Bio:

_____

_____

_____

_____

Client's Bio:

_____

_____

_____

_____

Caregiver's Bio:

_____

_____

_____

_____

Client's Bio:

_____

_____

_____

_____

Pain

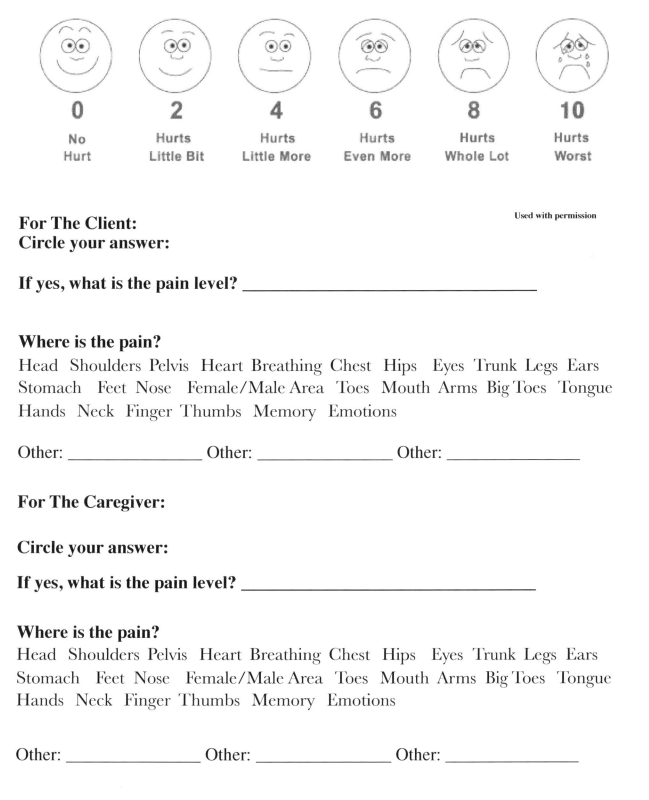

Wong-Baker FACES® Pain Rating Scale

0	2	4	6	8	10
No Hurt	Hurts Little Bit	Hurts Little More	Hurts Even More	Hurts Whole Lot	Hurts Worst

Used with permission

For The Client:
Circle your answer:

If yes, what is the pain level? _____

Where is the pain?

Head Shoulders Pelvis Heart Breathing Chest Hips Eyes Trunk Legs Ears
Stomach Feet Nose Female/Male Area Toes Mouth Arms Big Toes Tongue
Hands Neck Finger Thumbs Memory Emotions

Other: _____ Other: _____ Other: _____

For The Caregiver:

Circle your answer:

If yes, what is the pain level? _____

Where is the pain?

Head Shoulders Pelvis Heart Breathing Chest Hips Eyes Trunk Legs Ears
Stomach Feet Nose Female/Male Area Toes Mouth Arms Big Toes Tongue
Hands Neck Finger Thumbs Memory Emotions

Other: _____ Other: _____ Other: _____

Together, focus your energy on helping each other.

When we are in pain, we are heavy in our cells.

When we are not aware of what we are doing or how we are moving, we are heavy.

Pay attention to the pain you are having and see if you can decrease the level of intensity.

Breathe through the pain.

Don't hold your breath in feeling the pain.

Breathe.

Play

Play provides a space and an opportunity where the mind, the heart and the will can get together to relax, release, restore, regenerate, re-energize, rehabilitate, realign, revitalize and receive more fully the person who lives inside of you. Play creates an opportunity for healthier thought perceptions for form for any age or stage in life because of it's flexibility and freedom to be either structures or non-structures, linear or holistic.

In our nervous system, play represents itself as an open-ended communications' system that nourishes and builds upon internal and external processes in the areas of sensations, movement, learning, feeling, creating and relating. With play, we have the ability to reduce anxiety and stress because we involve ourselves in the present moment where there is an opportunity to relax, release, restore, regenerate, reenergize, rehabilitate, realign, revitalize and receive healthier perceptions of the evolving self.

Stress is reduced when we play and "let go" of tightness, tension and toxic waste build-up in the nervous system. With a laugh, a push or a pull, explore the curious possibilities of succeeds. Play lightens our load and makes us a more enjoyable person to be around.

Play is fun.

What do you consider to be fun and playful for you?

Client   **Caregiver**

_____   _____

_____   _____

_____   _____

_____   _____

_____   _____

_____   _____

_____   _____

_____   _____

_____   _____

Next time you have an opportunity, go to your neighborhood toy store because they typically have a great selection of toys and novelty items that are fun to explore.

Consider:

Tops

Whistles

Wind chimes

Jacks

Puzzles

Wands

Water snake

Tornado Tube

Pustfix Bear Bubbles

Heavenly Orb

Mini Finger Puppets

Putty or play-doh

Rainstick's

Flensted Mobiles

Wikki Stix

Jingle Bands

Drums

Magnetic Marbles

Marble Mazes

The Going

Slinky

Read To Each Other

Who read what, where, when.

Who Read: _____   **What** _____

Where: _____   **What Date:** _____

For How Long: _____   Experience Was: Positive Blah_____

Who Read: _____   **What** _____

Where: _____   **What Date:** _____

For How Long: _____   Experience Was: Positive Blah_____

Who Read: _____   **What** _____

Where: _____   **What Date:** _____

For How Long: _____   Experience Was: Positive Blah_____

Who Read: _____   **What** _____

Where: _____   **What Date:** _____

For How Long: _____   Experience Was: Positive Blah_____

Who Read: _____   **What** _____

Where: _____   **What Date:** _____

For How Long: _____   Experience Was: Positive Blah_____

Who Read: _____   **What** _____

Where: _____   **What Date:** _____

For How Long: _____   Experience Was: Positive Blah_____

Who Read: _____   **What** _____

Where: _____   **What Date:** _____

For How Long: _____   Experience Was: Positive Blah_____

Who Read: _____   **What** _____

Where: _____   **What Date:** _____

For How Long: _____   Experience Was: Positive Blah_____

Who Read: _____   **What** _____

Where: _____   **What Date:** _____

For How Long: _____   Experience Was: Positive Blah_____

Who Read: _____   **What** _____

Where: _____   **What Date:** _____

For How Long: _____   Experience Was: Positive Blah_____

Who Read: _____   **What** _____

Where: _____   **What Date:** _____

For How Long: _____   Experience Was: Positive Blah_____

Routines

Routines help us cope with life.

Client: Name a daily routine   Name a weekly routine

_____   _____

Would you like to change it?   Yes No   If yes, how? _____

_____

Routines help us cope with life.

Caregiver: Name a daily routine   Name a weekly routine

_____   _____

Would you like to change it?   Yes No   If yes, how? _____

_____

Routines help us cope with life.

Client: Name a daily routine   Name a weekly routine

_____   _____

Would you like to change it?   Yes No   If yes, how? _____

_____

Routines help us cope with life.

Caregiver: Name a daily routine   Name a weekly routine

_____   _____

Would you like to change it?   Yes No   If yes, how? _____

_____

Routines

Routines help us cope with life.

Client: Name a daily routine   Name a weekly routine

_____   _____

Would you like to change it?   Yes No   If yes, how? _____

_____

Routines help us cope with life.

Caregiver: Name a daily routine   Name a weekly routine

_____   _____

Would you like to change it?   Yes No   If yes, how? _____

_____

Routines help us cope with life.

Client: Name a daily routine   Name a weekly routine

_____   _____

Would you like to change it?   Yes No   If yes, how? _____

_____

Routines help us cope with life.

Caregiver: Name a daily routine   Name a weekly routine

_____   _____

Would you like to change it?   Yes No   If yes, how? _____

_____

Smell

It's a powerful connector to memory.

Explore

Client: **Favorite Smells**   **Smells that cause a negative reaction/how**

_____

_____

_____

_____

_____

_____

Caregiver: **Favorite Smells**   **Smells that cause a negative reaction/how**

_____

_____

_____

_____

_____

_____

Client: **Favorite Smells**   **Smells that cause a negative reaction/how**

_____

_____

_____

_____

_____

_____

Caregiver: **Favorite Smells**   **Smells that cause a negative reaction/how**

_____

_____

_____

_____

_____

_____

Start Your Story

"From the beginning of the human race stories have been used - by priests, by bards, by medicine men — as magic instruments of healing, of teaching, as a means of helping people come to terms with the fact that they continually have to face insoluble problems and unbearable realities."

- Joan Aiken

Lesson One

Three to Five Descriptive Words to start talking about your story.

Client

1._____

2._____

3._____

4._____

5._____

Caregiver

1._____

2._____

3._____

4._____

5._____

Start Your Story

Lesson Two

A. Circle three that match your story TODAY or the story you want to have.

B. Repeat these words as your story at least 10 to 50x's a day

_____, _____._____.

Caregiver	**Client**
Balance	Balance
Compassion	Compassion
Courage	Courage
Direction	Direction
Faith	Faith
Freedom	Freedom
Friendship	Friendship
Guardian	Guardian
Happy	Happy
Harmony	Harmony
Health	Health
Humility	Humility
Joy	Joy
Life	Life
Love	Love
Magic	Magic
Passion	Passion
Patience	Patience
Peace	Peace
Perseverance	Perseverance
Play	Play

Power	Power
Prosperity	Prosperity
Relationship	Relationship
Respect	Respect
Serenity	Serenity
Spirit	Spirit
Strength	Strength
Surrender	Surrender
Transformation	Transformation
Trust	Trust
Truth	Truth
Unity	Unity
Wisdom	Wisdom

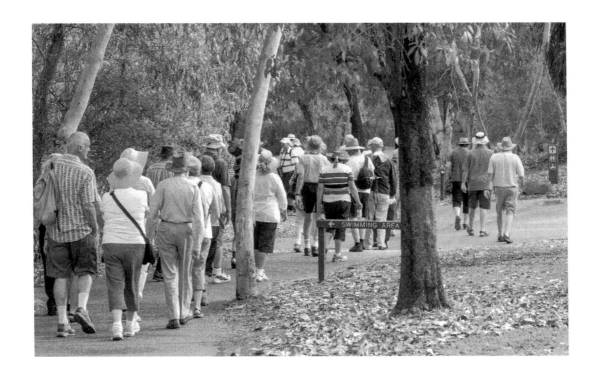

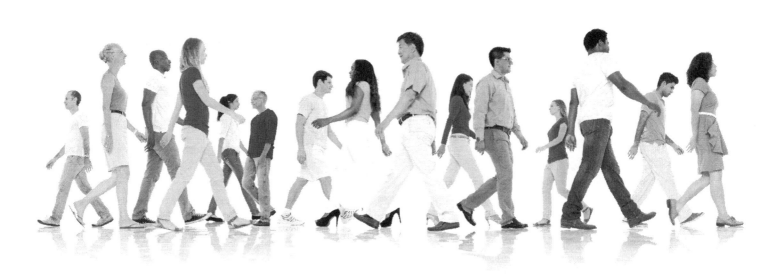

Walk

Do it together, a little bit every day.

Daily Walks

Day:_____ How Long_____ Where_____

Day:_____ How Long_____ Where_____

Day:_____ How Long_____ Where_____

Day:_____ How Long_____ Where_____

Day:_____ How Long_____ Where_____

Day:_____ How Long_____ Where_____

Day:_____ How Long_____ Where_____

Day:_____ How Long_____ Where_____

Day:_____ How Long_____ Where_____

Day:_____ How Long_____ Where_____

Day:_____ How Long_____ Where_____

Day:_____ How Long_____ Where_____

Day:_____ How Long_____ Where_____

Day:_____ How Long_____ Where_____

Day:_____ How Long_____ Where_____

Day:_____ How Long_____ Where_____

Day:_____ How Long_____ Where_____

Day:_____ How Long_____ Where_____

Day:_____ How Long_____ Where_____

Day:_____ **How Long**_____ **Where**_____

Day:_____ **How Long**_____ **Where**_____

Day:_____ **How Long**_____ **Where**_____

Day:_____ **How Long**_____ **Where**_____

Day:_____ **How Long**_____ **Where**_____

Day:_____ **How Long**_____ **Where**_____

Day:_____ **How Long**_____ **Where**_____

Day:_____ **How Long**_____ **Where**_____

Day:_____ **How Long**_____ **Where**_____

Day:_____ **How Long**_____ **Where**_____

Day:_____ **How Long**_____ **Where**_____

Day:_____ **How Long**_____ **Where**_____

Day:_____ **How Long**_____ **Where**_____

Day:_____ **How Long**_____ **Where**_____

Day:_____ **How Long**_____ **Where**_____

Day:_____ **How Long**_____ **Where**_____

Day:_____ **How Long**_____ **Where**_____

Day:_____ **How Long**_____ **Where**_____

Day:_____ **How Long**_____ **Where**_____

Day:_____ **How Long**_____ **Where**_____

Day:_____ **How Long**_____ **Where**_____

What Motivates You?

Physiological	Safety Security Of:	Love/Belonging	Esteem	Self-Actualization
Breathing	Body	Friendship	Self-Esteem	Morality
Food	Employment	Family	Confidence	Creativity
Water	Resources	Sexual Intimacy	Achievement	Spontaneity
Sex	Morality		Respect of Others	Problem Solving
Sleep	The Family		Respect by Others	Lack of Prejudice
Homeostasis	Health			Acceptance of Fact
Excretion	Property			

Lesson One:

Name The Three Top Sub-Categories That You Are Most Motivated By

Client	Caregiver
_____	_____
_____	_____
_____	_____

Discuss the similarities and the differences.

How can you work together?

A Plan To Work Together:

_____

_____

_____

Lesson Two:

Revisit These Motivations To See if Your Plan To Work Together Still Works.

Physiological	Safety Security Of:	Love/Belonging	Esteem	Self-Actualization
Breathing	Body	Friendship	Self-Esteem	Morality
Food	Employment	Family	Confidence	Creativity
Water	Resources	Sexual Intimacy	Achievement	Spontaneity
Sex	Morality		Respect of Others	Problem Solving
Sleep	The Family		Respect by Others	Lack of Prejudice
Homeostasis	Health			Acceptance of Fact
Excretion	Property			

Name The Three Top Sub-Categories That You Are Most Motivated By

Client	**Caregiver**
_____	_____
_____	_____
_____	_____

This is how you are driven.

Discuss the similarities and the differences.

How can you work together?

A Plan To Work Together:

_____

_____

_____

What Is Your Story For The Day?

(Write out a short paragraph about who you are today and then we will read what we have written to each other).

Client

_____

_____

_____

_____

_____

Caregiver:

_____

_____

_____

_____

Let's Read our story to one another now.

What did we find out about today from each other?

Caregiver with Client's Story:

_____

_____

Client with Caregiver's Story:

_____

_____

(Write out a short paragraph about who you are today and then we will read what we have written to each other).

Client

_____

_____

_____

_____

_____

Caregiver:

_____

_____

_____

_____

_____

Let's Read our story to one another now.

What did we find out about today from each other?

Caregiver with Client's Story:

_____

_____

Client with Caregiver's Story:

_____

_____

Whole Brain Involvement

We learn by using the whole brain with respect to our logical, linear, imaginative, intuitive, artistic, mathematical, scientific and musical capabilities, body awareness, auditory sequencing, visual perceptual sequencing, motor planning, memory, stress levels and individual adaptability. Everything influences whole brain thinking.

Understand More Of Yourself By Involving Yourself With Your Brain & Your Memory.

Lesson One: What Ways Do You Learn The Best?

Client:

_____

_____

_____

_____

_____

Caregiver:

_____

_____

_____

_____

_____

Lesson Two: Where Is Your Best Memory Found?

Like mathematical formulas, languages, dates and times, recipes, sports, emotional, music, etc…

Client	**Caregiver**
_____	_____
_____	_____
_____	_____

Lesson Three:

Now let's see how well you can remember what went on today. Name 3 things that stick out for you in your memory.

Client

1._____

2._____

3._____

Caregiver

1._____

2._____

3._____

Lesson Four:

How well can you remember what went on last week. Name 3 things that stick out for you in your memory.

Client

1._____

2._____

3._____

Caregiver

1._____

2._____

3._____

When I Get Mad I Talk to My Hand

This saves time and energy in everything. It is okay to get angry. Just diffuse by talking to your hand. When you are through, clap or shake your hands to get rid of that emotion. Wash your hands and know it's a new beginning.

Client	**Caregiver**
Day_____ Time_____Over - Yes/No	**Day**_____ Time_____Over - Yes/No
Day_____ Time_____Over - Yes/No	**Day**_____ Time_____Over - Yes/No
Day_____ Time_____Over - Yes/No	**Day**_____ Time_____Over - Yes/No
Day_____ Time_____Over - Yes/No	**Day**_____ Time_____Over - Yes/No
Day_____ Time_____Over - Yes/No	**Day**_____ Time_____Over - Yes/No
Day_____ Time_____Over - Yes/No	**Day**_____ Time_____Over - Yes/No
Day_____ Time_____Over - Yes/No	**Day**_____ Time_____Over - Yes/No
Day_____ Time_____Over - Yes/No	**Day**_____ Time_____Over - Yes/No
Day_____ Time_____Over - Yes/No	**Day**_____ Time_____Over - Yes/No
Day_____ Time_____Over - Yes/No	**Day**_____ Time_____Over - Yes/No
Day_____ Time_____Over - Yes/No	**Day**_____ Time_____Over - Yes/No
Day_____ Time_____Over - Yes/No	**Day**_____ Time_____Over - Yes/No
Day_____ Time_____Over - Yes/No	**Day**_____ Time_____Over - Yes/No
Day Time Over - Yes/No	**Day** Time Over - Yes/No

Client		**Caregiver**	

Day_____ Time_____Over - Yes/No   **Day**_____ Time_____Over - Yes/No

Day_____ Time_____Over - Yes/No   **Day**_____ Time_____Over - Yes/No

Day_____ Time_____Over - Yes/No   **Day**_____ Time_____Over - Yes/No

Day_____ Time_____Over - Yes/No   **Day**_____ Time_____Over - Yes/No

Day_____ Time_____Over - Yes/No   **Day**_____ Time_____Over - Yes/No

Day_____ Time_____Over - Yes/No   **Day**_____ Time_____Over - Yes/No

Day_____ Time_____Over - Yes/No   **Day**_____ Time_____Over - Yes/No

Day_____ Time_____Over - Yes/No   **Day**_____ Time_____Over - Yes/No

Day_____ Time_____Over - Yes/No   **Day**_____ Time_____Over - Yes/No

Day_____ Time_____Over - Yes/No   **Day**_____ Time_____Over - Yes/No

Day_____ Time_____Over - Yes/No   **Day**_____ Time_____Over - Yes/No

Day_____ Time_____Over - Yes/No   **Day**_____ Time_____Over - Yes/No

Day_____ Time_____Over - Yes/No   **Day**_____ Time_____Over - Yes/No

Day_____ Time_____Over - Yes/No   **Day**_____ Time_____Over - Yes/No

Day_____ Time_____Over - Yes/No   **Day**_____ Time_____Over - Yes/No

Day_____ Time_____Over - Yes/No   **Day**_____ Time_____Over - Yes/No

Day_____ Time_____Over - Yes/No   **Day**_____ Time_____Over - Yes/No

Day_____ Time_____Over - Yes/No   **Day**_____ Time_____Over - Yes/No

Writing Poems

Poems express our feelings and emotions in a condensed and centered way. This creative expression allows us to see our situation in a different way.

Here's some examples.

1). A poem that is in the shape it's describing.

My writing From "Points of Consciousness From The Camino" by Beth Lord

a
tear
is a fear
or a loving
care to feel
& release
Beth

Lesson One: Write a poem in a shape that it's about.
Client

Lesson One: Write a poem in a shape that it's about.

Caregiver

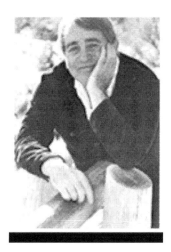

James Kavanaugh was a prolific and amazing writer.

"In a writing career that spanned forty years, Mr. Kavanaugh has been as prolific as he had been profound. He has published twenty-six books of philosophy, psychology, theology, fiction and poetry. Speaking of him, Wayne Dyer says: 'I can think of no living person who can put into words what we have all felt so deeply in our inner selves…'

http://www.jameskavanaugh.org

UNAFRAID TO BE FREE

Finally unafraid to be free,
Ready to surrender all the illusions of
recognition and external securities,
Living off the sky and earth like starting
eagles and braying burros,
Trusting in a Power even beyond Dow Jones
and hoarded retirement.
Finally ready to live like the noble animal that I am-
Without masters or servants, with dignity dependent on no one,
Content to know that I am God's child, and
only good has been prepared for me.
When I am not afraid to release all that my life
and culture taught me to prize.
To abandon fears once and for all, to discard the
anxieties of a lifetime like a suit that no longer fits,
To be afraid of no one, beholden to no one,
dependent on no one
Save the few who know and love me as I am,
and the God Who alone gives meaning and joy

Lesson Two: Write A Self-Reflective Poem

Client

Caregiver

Lesson Three:

Caregiver: Do you have a favorite poet?   **Yes**   **No**

             If yes, who is it _____

Client: **Do you have a favorite poet?**   **Yes**   **No**

             If yes, who is it _____

If not, here are some web-sites to explore. If you find a poet you like you can always take a trip to the library and see if they have any of their books to check out. If you don't have a library card, that would be another good activity to invest in.

http://famouspoetsandpoems.com

http://www.poets.org

http://www.familyfriendpoems.com/poems/famous/

http://allpoetry.com

http://www.poetryfoundation.org

http://www.poetry.org

http://www.poemhunter.com

http://www.famous-poems.biz/Short_Poems/Famous-Short-Poems-best-free-poetry-online.html

http://www.humorouspoems.net

http://www.funny-poems.biz

Lesson Four: Try to write a poem that rhymes.

Client

Caregiver

You Matter

Lesson One:

Write down people or pets you matter to.

Client	**Caregiver**
1. Yourself	**1. Yourself**_____
2. _____	2. _____
3. _____	3. _____
4. _____	4. _____
5. _____	5. _____
6. _____	6. _____
7. _____	7. _____
8. _____	8. _____
9. _____	9. _____
10. _____	10. _____
11. _____	11. _____
12. _____	12. _____
13. _____	13. _____
14. _____	14. _____
15. _____	15. _____

You Matter

Lesson Two:

Write down why.

Client	**Caregiver**
1. Because I am amazing.	**1. Because I am amazing.**
2. _____	2. _____
3. _____	3. _____
4. _____	4. _____
5. _____	5. _____
6. _____	6. _____
7. _____	7. _____
8. _____	8. _____
9. _____	9. _____
10. _____	10. _____
11. _____	11. _____
12. _____	12. _____
13. _____	13. _____
14. _____	14. _____
15. _____	15. _____

ABOUT THE AUTHOR

Beth is a writer, therapist & healer in helping you remember your story and stories that mean the most to you in your write heart memories®. She listens to you and turns your stories into books for you.

Go To Beth's Website:www.bethlord.com
Like Beth On Facebook
Download Beth's free ebooks.
Subscribe to Beth's blog.
Subscribe to Beth's newsletter.
Send Beth an email atbeth@bethlord.com
Give Beth a call at 206.498.2532
On Instagram as writeheartmemories.

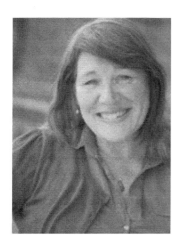

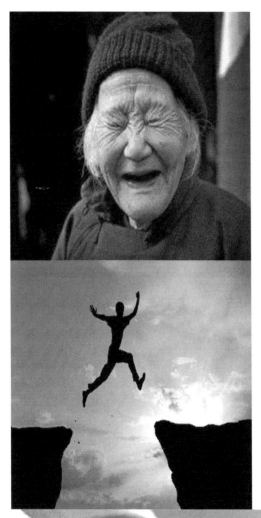

We Are Amazing!

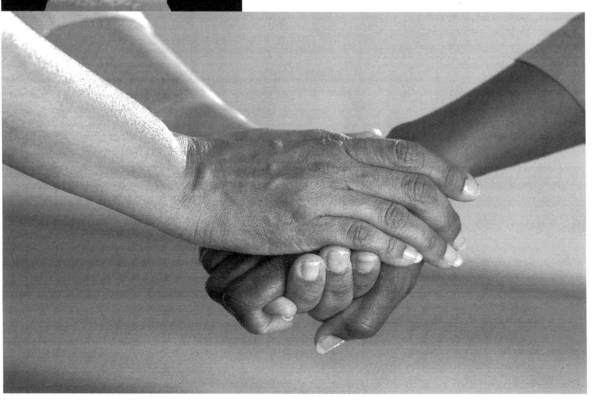

Made in the USA
San Bernardino, CA
17 March 2016